Chronic Traumatic Encephalopathy

Proceedings of the Boston University Alzheimer's Disease Center Conference

Chronic Traumatic Encephalopathy

Proceedings of the Boston University Alzheimer's Disease Center Conference

ANDREW E. BUDSON, MD
Section Chief, Cognitive & Behavioral
  Neurology
Associate Chief of Staff for Education
Veterans Affairs Boston Healthcare System
Associate Director and Education Core
  Director, Boston University Alzheimer's
  Disease Center
Professor of Neurology
Boston University School of Medicine
Lecturer in Neurology and Academy
  Member
Harvard Medical School
Boston, MA

ANN C. MCKEE, MD
Chief of Neuropathology Service
Veterans Affairs Boston Healthcare System
Associate Director and Neuropathology
  Core Director, Boston University
  Alzheimer's Disease Center
Professor of Neurology and Pathology
Boston University School of Medicine
Boston, MA

ROBERT C. CANTU, MA, MD,
FACS, FACSM, FAANS
Clinical Professor of Neurosurgery and
  Neurology, and Clinical Diagnostics and
  Therapeutics Leader, Alzheimer's Disease
  Center
Boston University School of Medicine
Boston, MA;
Associate Chair, Department of Surgery
Chief, Neurosurgery Service
Director of Sports Medicine
Emerson Hospital
Concord, MA

ROBERT A. STERN, PhD
Professor of Neurology, Neurosurgery, and
  Anatomy & Neurobiology
Boston University School of Medicine
Clinical Core Director, Boston University
  Alzheimer's Disease and Chronic
  Traumatic Encephalopathy Centers
Boston, MA

ELSEVIER

ELSEVIER

1600 John F. Kennedy Blvd.
Ste 1800
Philadelphia, PA 19103-2899

CHRONIC TRAUMATIC ENCEPHALOPATHY: PROCEEDINGS OF THE
BOSTON UNIVERSITY ALZHEIMER'S DISEASE CENTER CONFERENCE   ISBN: 978-0-323-54425-2

Content Strategist: Kayla Wolfe
Design Direction: Renee Duenow

Working together
to grow libraries in
developing countries

www.elsevier.com • www.bookaid.org

Contributors

Bobak Abdolmohammadi, BA
Research Assistant
Boston University Chronic Traumatic Encephalopathy
    Center
Boston, MA

Michael L. Alosco, PhD
NRSA Postdoctoral Fellow
Boston University Alzheimer's Disease and Chronic
    Traumatic Encephalopathy Centers
Boston University School of Medicine
Boston, MA

Victor E. Alvarez, MD
Assistant Professor of Neurology
Boston University School of Medicine
Physician Research Associate
Boston University Alzheimer's Disease and Chronic
    Traumatic Encephalopathy Centers
PTSD Brain Bank
Veterans Affairs Boston Healthcare System
Boston, MA

Franck Amyot, PhD
Department of Neurology
Center for Neuroscience and Regenerative Medicine
Uniformed Services University of the Health
    Sciences
Bethesda, MD

Kaj Blennow, MD, PhD
Professor and Academic Chair
Clinical Neurochemistry Laboratory
Institute of Neuroscience and Physiology
The Sahlgrenska Academy at Gothenburg University
Gothenburg, Sweden;
The Söderberg Professorship in Medicine
The Royal Academy of Science
Stockholm, Sweden

Andrew E. Budson, MD
Section Chief, Cognitive & Behavioral Neurology and
Associate Chief of Staff for Education
Veterans Affairs Boston Healthcare System
Associate Director and Education Core Director
Boston University Alzheimer's Disease Center
Professor of Neurology
Boston University School of Medicine
Lecturer in Neurology and Academy Member
Harvard Medical School
Boston, MA

Robert C. Cantu, MA, MD, FACS, FACSM, FAANS
Clinical Professor of Neurosurgery and Neurology,
    and Clinical Diagnostics and Therapeutics Leader,
    Alzheimer's Disease Center, Boston University
    School of Medicine
Senior Advisor, Brain Injury Center, Children's
    Hospital
Boston, MA;
Medical Director and Director of Clinical Research,
    Dr. Robert C. Cantu Concussion Center
Associate Chair, Department of Surgery
Chief, Neurosurgery Service
Director of Sports Medicine
Emerson Hospital
Concord, MA;
Medical Director, National Center for Catastrophic
    Sports Injury Research
Co-Founder, Medical Director, Concussion Legacy
    Foundation
Senior Advisor, NFL Head, Neck, & Spine
    Committee
Clinical Advisor, NFL Engineering Sub-Committee
Member, NFLPA Mackey-White Player Health and
    Safety Committee
Senior Advisor, National Council Youth Sports
    Safety
Member, Concussion Advisory Group, World
    Rugby

Ramon Diaz-Arrastia, MD, PhD
Department of Neurology
Penn Center for Brain Injury and Repair
University of Pennsylvania Perelman School of
    Medicine
Philadelphia, PA

Thomas A. Gennarelli, MD
Emeritus Professor of Neurosurgery
Medical College of Wisconsin
Clinical Professor of Neurosurgery
George Washington University
Washington, DC

Lee Goldstein, MD, PhD
Associate Professor in Psychiatry, Neurology,
    Ophthalmology, Pathology and Laboratory
    Medicine, Biomedical Engineering, Electrical &
    Computer Engineering.
College of Engineering, Photonics Center
Boston University School of Medicine
Translational and Discovery Core Leader, Boston
    University Alzheimer's Disease Center
Investigator, Chronic Traumatic Encephalopathy
    Center
Boston, MA

Margalit Haber, PhD
Department of Neurology
Penn Center for Brain Injury and Repair
University of Pennsylvania Perelman School of Medicine
Philadelphia, PA

Bertrand R. Huber, MD, PhD
Director, PTSD Brain Bank
Veterans Affairs Boston Healthcare System
Assistant Professor of Neurology
Boston University School of Medicine
Neuropathologist, Neuropathology Core, Boston
    University Alzheimer's Disease and Chronic
    Traumatic Encephalopathy Centers
Boston, MA

Kimbra Kenney, MD
Department of Neurology
Center for Neuroscience and Regenerative Medicine
Uniformed Services University of the Health
    Sciences
Bethesda, MD

Inga K. Koerte, MD
Department of Psychiatry
Brigham and Women's Hospital and Harvard Medical
    School
Boston, MA;
Department of Child and Adolescent Psychiatry,
    Psychosomatics, and Psychotherapy
Ludwig-Maximilians-Universität
Munich, Germany

Ann C. McKee, MD
Chief of Neuropathology Service
Veterans Affairs Boston Healthcare System
Director, Chronic Traumatic Encephalopathy Center
Associate Director and Neuropathology Core Director,
    Boston University Alzheimer's Disease Center
Professor of Neurology and Pathology
Boston University School of Medicine
Boston, MA

Jesse Mez, MD, MS
Assistant Professor of Neurology
Boston University School of Medicine
Clinical Core Associate Director
Boston University Alzheimer's Disease and Chronic
    Traumatic Encephalopathy Centers
Boston, MA

Carol Moore, MA
Department of Neurology
Penn Center for Brain Injury and Repair
University of Pennsylvania Perelman School of
    Medicine
Philadelphia, PA

Christopher J. Nowinski, AB, PhD
Co-Founder & CEO, Concussion Legacy
    Foundation
Outreach, Recruitment, Education, and Public Policy
    Leader
Boston University Alzheimer's Disease and Chronic
    Traumatic Encephalopathy Centers
Boston, MA

Bethany Rowson, DVM, PhD
Department of Biomedical Engineering and
    Mechanics
Virginia Tech
Blacksburg, VA

Steven Rowson, PhD
Department of Biomedical Engineering and Mechanics
Virginia Tech
Blacksburg, VA

Martha E. Shenton, PhD
Research and Development
Veterans Affairs Boston Healthcare System
Departments of Psychiatry and Radiology
Brigham and Women's Hospital and Harvard Medical
    School
Boston, MA

Thor D. Stein, MD, PhD
Neuropathology Core Associate Director
Boston University Alzheimer's Disease and Chronic
    Traumatic Encephalopathy Centers
Assistant Professor of Pathology and Laboratory
    Medicine
Boston University School of Medicine
Neuropathologist
Veterans Affairs Boston Healthcare System and Edith
    Nourse Rogers Memorial Veterans Hospital
Boston, MA

Robert A. Stern, PhD
Professor of Neurology, Neurosurgery, and
    Anatomy & Neurobiology
Boston University School of Medicine
Clinical Core Director, Boston University Alzheimer's
    Disease and Chronic Traumatic Encephalopathy
    Centers
Boston, MA

Foreword

The opportunity to witness the rediscovery and reinvention of a disease is a rare experience. Alzheimer's disease (AD) was first described in 1906 but sat on the back burner for 70 years until Bob Katzman and Bob Terry rediscovered and reinvented it. Since then the pace and intensity of AD research and discovery have grown exponentially. I believe we are now privileged to be witnessing a similar transformation in our understanding of the "punch drunk" syndrome or dementia pugilistica, first described by Martland over 80 years ago. Ann McKee, chief of neuropathology at the Veterans Affairs Boston Healthcare System, director of the Boston University Chronic Traumatic Encephalopathy (BU CTE) Center, and director of the neuropathology core of the Boston University Alzheimer's Disease Center (BU ADC); Robert Stern, director of the clinical cores of the BU ADC and the BU CTE Center; and their colleagues at BU and around the country have truly reinvented this disease, now best known as chronic traumatic encephalopathy (CTE), the name given by Sir Macdonald Critchley in the 1950s. Ann McKee's landmark postmortem studies over the past 8 years have defined and refined the diagnostic features and neuropathologic staging of CTE and established it as a unique acquired tauopathy distinguishable from other neurodegenerative diseases. She has amassed the world's largest collection of postmortem CTE brains, many of which were donated by the families of retired National Football League players. Interest and awareness of CTE have been amplified in the public eye through the mainstream media. The pace of CTE research has begun to accelerate and catch up with the publicity. Ann McKee and Bob Stern are leading large national multisite programs, funded by the Department of Veterans Affairs, the National Institutes of Health, and the Department of Defense, to better understand the diagnostic and clinical features of CTE. Their clinical pathologic correlation studies and clinical observations of athletes exposed to high levels of repetitive head impact are driving the formulation of key research questions that will likely fuel an explosion of new CTE research and discovery. Because of this rapid progress, the leadership of the BU ADC felt that the time was right to sponsor a symposium bringing together leaders in the field of CTE research to present their current work and near-term future plans, including unpublished data and new ideas. This volume is a transcribed and edited summary of the symposium held at Boston University in November 2016. In these proceedings Drs. McKee and Stern summarize their current work on CTE neuropathology and clinical features. Thor Stein, a neuropathology colleague of Ann McKee's, presents new data regarding comorbid pathology in CTE brains. Martha Shenton, an expert on brain imaging, presents her work on magnetic resonance imaging of athletes. Jesse Mez, a neurologist and statistical geneticist at BU, discusses what is known about CTE genetics and where the field is going. Bob Cantu, a distinguished senior clinician and leader in the field with over 50 years of clinical experience, reviews the history of concussion and CTE research. Andrew Budson, a practicing behavioral neurologist, educator, and investigator, outlines a practical approach to the differential diagnosis and symptomatic treatment of CTE and other causes of progressive cognitive decline in the clinic. Kaj Blennow, an international expert on neurodegenerative disease biomarkers, presents exciting new data on potential CTE biomarkers. Ramon Diaz-Arrastia, a neurologist and leader in therapeutic trials for traumatic brain injury, presents an approach to CTE clinical trials and therapeutics. Lee Goldstein, director of the BU Molecular Aging and Development Laboratory, has developed remarkable mouse models of blast injury and concussion that are illuminating mechanisms of neuronal injury in CTE. Steve and Bethany Rowson, engineers who study brain injury biomechanics, present an update on what is currently known about the biomechanics of head injury. A unique feature of this volume is the inclusion of two special chapters. Chris Nowinski, cofounder and CEO of the Concussion Legacy Foundation and a retired professional wrestler, led a discussion with three high-profile professional athletes who are suffering from the effects of chronic repetitive head impacts. Their reflections and perspectives as players give us a first-person window into the consequences of extensive exposure to repeated head impacts and perceptive insights into what might be done to mitigate risks for the next generation of athletes. Bob Stern led a discussion with family members that will move readers to further appreciate the tragic repercussions of CTE and how it affects both individuals and their loved ones. I am confident that investigators studying traumatic brain injury and neurodegenerative diseases, clinicians caring for patients who have sustained repetitive head injuries, and others interested in the field will find this timely volume both informative and useful.

Neil Kowall, MD
Professor of Neurology and Pathology
Boston University School of Medicine
Director, Boston University Alzheimer's Disease Center
Chief, Neurology Service, Veterans Affairs Boston
Healthcare System

Preface

This book contains the proceedings of the Boston University Alzheimer's Disease Center Conference on Chronic Traumatic Encephalopathy (CTE) held at Boston University, November 3 and 4, 2016. It provides an up-to-date reference of the basic and clinical science of CTE and how we care for patients with presumed CTE in our practices. It also gives a glimpse into the human side of this disorder by presenting interviews with former football players and boxers, as well as with family members of individuals who died with CTE.

The presenters at our 2-day conference showed much enthusiasm for their work, hoping that it may provide a better understanding of this disorder today and lead to possible treatment and prevention of the disorder in the future. What follows in these pages are chapters created from actual transcripts of the conference lectures. Although the transcripts have been heavily edited to form easy-to-read chapters, we have purposely retained the speakers' enthusiasm and colloquial use of language. We found that keeping some of the lecturers' style has made the book particularly accessible, whether you read it cover to cover as our participants experienced the conference or you choose particular chapters that are of interest to you. In either case, we hope that you will be able to hear the presenters speak to you through these pages.

CTE is a devastating disorder that damages and sometimes destroys individuals and families. Thanks to the leading-edge research being conducted, however, there is hope for the future for those who are at risk for this disorder and for their families. Whether you are a clinician, scientist, or someone touched by the disease, we believe that you will find valuable information within these pages.

Andrew E. Budson, MD
Ann C. McKee, MD
Robert C. Cantu, MD
Robert A. Stern, PhD
Boston, Massachusetts

Acknowledgments

This book is dedicated to all of those who have experienced the difficulties of chronic traumatic encephalopathy, especially individuals with the disorder, their families, and their friends.

The contributions of many people were critical for the success of this book and the conference that preceded it, but none more so than that of Ms. Christina DiTerlizzi. We wish to give her our special thanks.

The content of this book has been derived from patients who were seen and research that was conducted outside of the VA Boston Healthcare system, along with literature reviews conducted solely for the purpose of this book. These reviews and the writing of this book have been conducted outside of the VA tours of duty of Drs. Budson, McKee, Stein, and Kowall. Note that 100% of the proceeds of this book are donated to the Education Core of the Boston University Alzheimer's Disease Center.

Contents

CHAPTER 1

History of Concussion and Chronic Traumatic Encephalopathy

ROBERT C. CANTU • THOMAS A. GENNARELLI

INTRODUCTION

Good morning everyone. I guess they have given the oldest person the task of leading off. I will be giving you some history. It is fun for me to be giving this talk because I have lived an awful lot of this history—about 50 plus years in terms of the concussion part of it and a fair amount in regards to the chronic traumatic encephalopathy (CTE) part, which is now being remade by Dr. Ann McKee, Dr. Robert Stern, and the Boston University (BU) group. We are all so thrilled to be a part of this history.

Let me start with a question. How many people think this statement is true: "Today there are more concussions occurring because players are bigger, stronger, and faster"? Or is it that, "There are more concussions today because we are better at recognizing concussions and documenting them"? How many people would think that's true? How many of you think both of these statements are true? How many people think there is even more to it? I am going to circle back to these questions in a little bit.

HISTORICAL THEORIES OF CONCUSSION

Going way back to the 1960s there were a number of theories about concussions. There was a vascular theory that the symptoms that occur after mechanically induced head trauma resulted from the constriction of blood flow to certain areas of the brain. The reticular theory—that the ascending reticular activating system (ARAS) was affected—was popular because prior to the mid-1970s virtually all concussions were diagnosed when there was loss of consciousness. We know that this system—running from the upper cervical cord at C1 up to the thalamus—is what is involved in the wakeful state. So that particular theory of concussion was held in pretty high regard at that point. Most concussions were not athletic concussions; they were mostly involving automobile accidents with high-speed trauma. So concussions at this time usually involved a loss of consciousness. There was a centripetal theory from Ommaya. There was the pontine cholinergic system theory. There were also other theories that, way back in the day 50 plus years ago, had some series advocates. One was related to the fact that after a concussive event and loss of consciousness there is very often what we now believe is a brainstem reflex, and that is abnormal posturing of the athlete with stiffening of their legs and bringing their arms up. This posture isn't due to a seizure, and we really believe that it is more of a brainstem reflex. Over the years it hasn't been correlated with the severity of concussion, but way back in the day, people thought it was.

Theories of Concussion
- Vascular: brief ischemia, decreased cerebral blood flow
- Reticular: brainstem site, effect on the ARAS produces loss of consciousness
- Centripetal: a complex variation of reticular
- Pontine cholinergic system: activation of the inhibitory system in the dorsal pons
- Convulsive: symptoms like those of a seizure

Definitions of Concussion
Prior to the mid-1970s, most physicians defined concussion as a loss of consciousness. Then in the mid-1970s into the 1980s concussion became more and more well recognized, and we understood that you don't have to be unconscious, you just need an alteration of the level of consciousness. So being stunned or concussed or having amnesia would get you into a concussed group without loss of consciousness. Then when we got further into the 1980s there were more and more symptoms of concussion. There were somatic symptoms, including light sensitivity, noise sensitivity, and headaches. There were also mood symptoms, behavior symptoms, and sleep symptoms—when they were traumatically induced, those nonspecific symptoms pretty much became the definition of concussion.

More recently, from the year 2000 onward, it has been pretty much any mechanically induced symptoms that have been used to define concussion.

Centripetal Theory of Concussion

In 1974, two neurosurgeons, Ayub Ommaya and Tom Gennarelli, wrote a seminal paper entitled, "Cerebral concussion and traumatic unconsciousness. Correlation of experimental and clinical observations of blunt head injuries." Published in the journal *Brain*, it presented the centripetal theory of concussion, many aspects of which have survived to this day. The concept that there are stresses and strains in the brain that are mechanically induced is really what we are working on today to better understand concussion. The centripetal theory also has a part that didn't stand the test of time; that was that mechanically induced forces would be maximal in the periphery of the brain, and if they were severe enough they would make their way down to the central parts of the brain to the brainstem itself.

Loss of Consciousness

In the late 1990s the American Academy of Neurology came out with their guidelines that suggested being unconscious was the only way to get you into the most severe grade of concussion. At the time they came out, people in the field quickly realized that these guidelines weren't really stacking up with what they were seeing in terms of how long patients' symptoms lasted, etc. There were then many consensus concussion guidelines that immediately came out countering the loss of consciousness requirement. Eventually, the American Academy of Neurology dropped those guidelines, but they were based on the centripetal theory, which has many components that have lived until today. But we are very much working today to understand and try to correlate the magnitude of the stresses and the strains and how their levels correlate with concussion. As of today we really don't have this relationship worked out. Just like we don't have thresholds for concussions in terms of the linear and acceleration forces that produce them, we don't really have the strain patterns that correlate with them as well.

Researchers of Concussions and Their Sequelae

It's fun for me to be a person who got involved in this field in terms of treating patients and diagnosing concussions back in the 1960s, and then athletic concussions from the 1970s through today (Fig. 1.1). Back when we first got involved, this was pretty much a field that involved neurosurgeons; it didn't really involve neurologists back then because it was trauma.

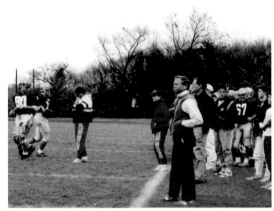

FIG. 1.1 A young Dr. Robert Cantu stands on the sidelines of a high school football game. (Image courtesy of Dr. Cantu.)

Then starting in the mid-1970s and going through to today, neurosurgeons remained an important part of the field but the neuroscientists, neurologists, neuropathologists, neuropsychologists, and many related disciplines became the majority of the people working in this field today. Today neuropathology is key, and we are going to hear from Dr. McKee about the importance of neuropathology to help us understand not just CTE but also concussion (Chapter 2). Neuropsychologists, neuroradiologists, and neuroscientists have more or less taken over a lot of this field today, and they are giving us wonderful contributions, improving our understanding.

CURRENT UNDERSTANDING OF CONCUSSION

Forces Needed to Produce Concussion

Let's reflect for a second on the question I posed about whether there are more concussions today or are we just recognizing more. Back in the day when concussion was defined as loss of consciousness, high forces were required to have a concussion because high forces were needed to produce that loss of consciousness. The mean acceleration force needed to produce loss of consciousness is approximately 6000 radians per second squared (Fig. 1.2). So back in the day when concussion was defined as loss of consciousness, the mean forces involved for most of those concussions were in that ballpark. Quite a high figure. As we started to redefine concussion, now there didn't need to be unconsciousness but just an alteration in the level of consciousness. So maybe the individual was stunned, foggy, or not taking in information. The forces needed to produce that alteration of consciousness were not as

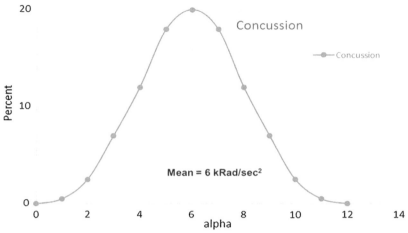

FIG. 1.2 Mean force needed to produce concussion before 1970, when concussion was defined as loss of consciousness. (Figure courtesy of Thomas Gennarelli.)

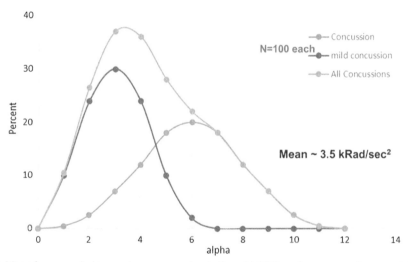

FIG. 1.3 Mean force needed to produce concussion in the mid-1970s, when concussion was defined as either mild, producing an alteration of consciousness, or more than mild, causing loss of consciousness. (Figure courtesy of Thomas Gennarelli.)

great, maybe around 3000 to 4000 radians per second squared (Fig. 1.3).

Current Definition of Concussion

The current definition of concussion is a traumatic brain injury caused by a bump, blow, or jolt to the head that can change the way your brain normally works. There can also be indirect loading of the brain with the inertia from whiplash or blast injury—the head does not have to be directly hit for the brain to be injured. The forces to produce symptoms may be even less, say 2 to 3 radians per second squared.

CONCUSSION IN ATHLETES

Grading the Severity of Concussions

My involvement with athletes started in the early 1970s when, as a younger neurosurgeon who was academically based at Massachusetts General Hospital and Boston City Hospital in terms of clinical practice, I moved with my young family to the suburbs, and I was suddenly thrust onto the sidelines of high school football teams as their team physician (Fig. 1.1). I realized that there was not a return-to-play guideline to help determine when those players who sustained a concussion should and shouldn't go back to playing football. We researched the literature, which was pretty slim at that point in time, and then wrote empirically based guidelines, as well as a grading system for concussion.[1]

The grading system was heavily influenced by what was being used in the mid-1980s, and so the mild grade involved no loss of consciousness and posttraumatic amnesia under 30 min, the moderate grade involved loss of consciousness under 5 min and posttraumatic amnesia greater in 30 min, and then the severe grade was loss of consciousness greater than 5 min, posttraumatic amnesia greater than 24 h.[1]

We realized through the years that having a grading scale without accounting for postconcussion symptoms was leaving out a very important component. We also found that, although 5 min was a commonly used amount of time for loss of consciousness when talking about concussions, a 5-min loss of consciousness was rarely observed on an athletic field. So in 2001 the criteria were upgraded based upon the duration of symptoms—the duration of abnormal brain activity (Box 1.1). So the grade 1 became no loss of consciousness and symptoms that cleared within 30 min. Back in the day, we were letting people go back to play whose symptoms rapidly did clear and you could not demonstrate additional symptoms after exerting them. Grade 2 was an individual who had a brief loss of consciousness, a greater duration of symptoms (but less than a week), and posttraumatic amnesia under 24 h. Grade 3 was an individual with a greater loss of consciousness, greater period of posttraumatic amnesia, and symptoms lasting greater than a week.[2]

BOX 1.1
Evidence-Based Cantu Revised Concussion-Grading Guidelines

- Grade 1 (mild): No loss of consciousness; posttraumatic amnesia/postconcussive signs and symptoms <30 min
- Grade 2 (moderate): Loss of consciousness <1 min or posttraumatic amnesia/postconcussive signs and symptoms >30 min
- Grade 3 (severe): Loss of consciousness ≥1 min or posttraumatic amnesia ≥24 h, postconcussive signs and symptoms >7 days

From Cantu RC. Posttraumatic Retrograde and Anterograde Amnesia: Pathophysiology and Implications in Grading and Safe Return to Play. *Journal of Athletic Training*. September 2001; 36(3):244–248. PMID: 12937491.

I think it is important to note that most definitions of concussion that others have developed are from severe concussions in individuals who had a prolonged loss of consciousness and other symptoms. Virtually all of the athletic concussions do not have loss of consciousness greater than a minute. In fact, loss of consciousness is present in less than 10% of the total athletic concussions, and when it does occur the loss of consciousness usually lasts just a few brief seconds. Many of the individuals in this 10% group with brief loss of consciousness do end up in the grade 3 (severe) category because their postconcussive symptoms often last more than a week.

Return-to-Play Guidelines

In those 1986 and 2001 papers the focus was really on return-to-play guidelines. Although they were empirically based at that time, it is worth noting that 30 years later we have the latest consensus statement from the International Concussion Conference in Berlin that I was just at, and the criteria are not much changed from 1986.

Thirty years ago, we felt that if you had a mild, grade 1 concussion where the symptoms cleared quickly, you could return to play if you were asymptomatic for a week (Table 1.1). Importantly, before you were allowed back you had to be not only asymptomatic at rest, you also had to be asymptomatic with exertion. So we had an exertion component built into the guidelines 30 years ago as there is today.

If individuals had a greater number of concussions or more severe concussions defined by a greater duration of symptoms, the period of time that they would be out of play was greater, as you can see from this grading system (Table 1.1). Grading systems are not necessary to manage a concussion. Grading systems ended up being eliminated from the consensus statements not because they weren't useful, but primarily because you don't absolutely need them. I would agree that you don't need a grading system, but it's very important, if you don't use one, that after you have evaluated the concussion, you describe how long the symptoms lasted. Although it may not be important whether it's a grade 2 or 3 concussion, it is important to understand the magnitude of the brain injury. Certainly a brain injury where symptoms last 3 weeks or 6 months is not the same injury where the symptoms have cleared within an hour or two. Table 1.2 shows the most recent published return-to-play protocol.[3]

Salient concussion position statements and grading scales:
- 1986 Cantu Return-to-Play Guidelines
- 1994 National Athletic Trainers' Association Summit
- 1996 American Academy of Neurology Grading Scale

TABLE 1.1
Guidelines for Return to Play After Concussion

	First Concussion	Second Concussion	Third Concussion
Grade 1 (mild)	May return to play if asymptomatic[a] for 1 wk	Return to play in 2 wk if asymptomatic at that time for 1 wk	Terminate season; may return to play next season if asymptomatic
Grade 2 (moderate)	Return to play after asymptomatic for 1 wk	Minimum of 1 mo; may return to play then if asymptomatic for 1 wk; consider terminating season	Terminate season; may return to play next season if asymptomatic
Grade 3 (severe)	Minimum of 1 mo; may then return to play if asymptomatic for 1 wk	Terminate season; may return to play next season if asymptomatic	

[a]No headache; dizziness, or impaired orientation, concentration, or memory during rest or exertion.
From Cantu RC. Guidelines for return to contact sports after a cerebral concussion. *The Physician and Sportsmedicine*. October 1986;14(10):75–83. http://dx.doi.org/10.1080/00913847.1986.11709197. PMID: 27432133

TABLE 1.2
Current Published Graduated Return-To-Play Protocol

Rehabilitation Stage	Functional Exercise at Each Stage of Rehabilitation	Objective of Each Stage
1. No activity	Symptom-limited physical and cognitive rest	Recovery
2. Light aerobic exercise	Walking, swimming, or stationary cycling keeping intensity <70% maximum permitted heart rate (HR) No resistance training	Increase HR
3. Sport-specific exercise	Skating drills in ice hockey, running drills in soccer No head impact activities	Add movement
4. Noncontact training drills	Progression to more complex training drills, e.g., passing drills in football and ice hockey May start progressive resistance training	Exercise, coordination, and cognitive load
5. Full-contact practice	Following medical clearance participate in normal training activities	Restore confidence and assess functional skills by coaching staff
6. Return to play	Normal game play	

From McCrory P, Meeuwisse WH, Aubry M, et al. Consensus statement on concussion in sport: the 4th International Conference on Concussion in Sport held in Zurich, November 2012. *British Journal of Sports Medicine*. April 2013; 47(5):250–258. http://dx.doi.org/10.1136/bjsports-2013-092313. PMID: 23479479

- 2001 Cantu Revised Grading Scale
- 2001 First International Concussion Conference (Vienna)
- 2004 National Athletic Trainers' Association Guidelines
- 2004 Second International Concussion Conference (Prague)
- 2006 American College of Sports Medicine Position Statement
- 2009 Third International Concussion Conference (Zurich)
- 2010 National Football League Guidelines
- 2011 Updated American College of Sports Medicine Position Statement

- 2012 Updated National Athletic Trainers' Association Guidelines
- 2012 National Football League Return-to-Play Guidelines
- 2012 Fourth International Concussion Conference (Zurich)
- 2016 Fifth International Concussion Conference (Berlin)

Through the years there have been a lot of consensus meetings and position statements put out by various organizations that we have been involved with. Although there has been wonderful participation, today we're still lacking the evidence needed to make the best decisions.

Toward a Definition of Concussion

To get back to the question about whether there are more concussions today because we are better at recognizing them or because players are bigger, faster, and stronger (or there is some other explanation), Fig. 1.4

shows the definition of concussion that is most prevalent today. When there is mechanical energy, acceleration, and rotational stresses imparted on the brain that result in altered brain function that leads to symptoms and signs, we recognize that as a concussion. But if there is no altered brain response, then there are no signs and symptoms, and we do not recognize that as a concussion.

I'll just mention now that in a seminal paper that I am sure Dr. Lee Goldstein will talk about (Chapter 5), we now understand that we can probably bypass concussion when we are trying to understand later life issues of neurodegeneration, CTE and the like, which are likely related not just to recognized concussions but also to the total brain trauma that has occurred. There is also other literature that discusses the structural, metabolic, and functional changes that occur with subconcussive blows to the head. Obviously, if we are talking about just the symptoms, they can occur with lesser stresses and lesser forces (Fig. 1.5).

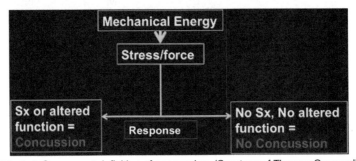

FIG. 1.4 One current definition of concussion. (Courtesy of Thomas Gennarelli.)

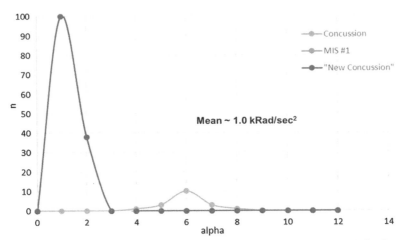

FIG. 1.5 Mean force needed to produce concussion after 2010, when concussion is defined as any mechanically induced symptom (*orange line*). *Gray line* shows prior concussion criteria related to loss of consciousness. (Figure courtesy of Thomas Gennarelli.)

So part of the answer to the question about whether we are recognizing concussions more is that we are really defining concussion in a new way. No longer is "concussion" the same as "cerebral concussion."[4,5] Many of the symptoms currently ascribed to concussion (or mild traumatic brain injury) are arguably not of cerebral or even brain origin. These symptoms include headache, dizziness, "seeing stars," tinnitus, fuzzy or blurred vision, fatigue, neck pain, photophobia, taste or smell disorders, sensitivity to noise, and others. We are really describing concussion as being related not only to movement of the brain, but also to factors that involve cranial nerves and cervical spine that can also produce symptoms as a result of head motion.

Additionally, when mechanically induced head motion affects the brain, it can affect various parts of the brain, including the neurons (axons, soma, dendrites, synapses, networks), blood vessels (arterial, venous, capillary) and possibly vasoconstriction or vasodilatation, oligodendrocytes (which can undergo demyelination causing altered electric transmission), astrocytes (causing gliosis), and microglia (causing inflammation). Keeping these different parts of the brain in mind is so important, and these different mechanisms are emerging as major factors not just in concussion but also in the later life consequences of concussion.

Mechanically Induced Concussion Symptoms

If we are using a symptoms-based definition of concussion, we need to think about what else besides the brain can actually be concussed by mechanical forces. You can have an olfactory concussion where the olfactory bulbs and tracks can be sheared and, as a result of that, you can have diminished (or rarely greater) smell (Fig. 1.6). The vestibular concussion or, more commonly, the vestibular symptoms of concussion, especially the peripheral vestibular symptoms, emanate from the semicircular canals and are transmitted by the vestibular portion of the eighth cranial nerve (Fig. 1.7). The cochlear portion of the nerve leads to the auditory system, in which greater sensitivity to noise is the most common symptom compared with decreased sensitivity (Fig. 1.7). Visual symptoms can be related to problems with smooth pursuit and eye movements controlled by our third, fourth, and sixth cranial nerves. Visual symptoms can also directly arise from injury to the retina itself, and so we can think

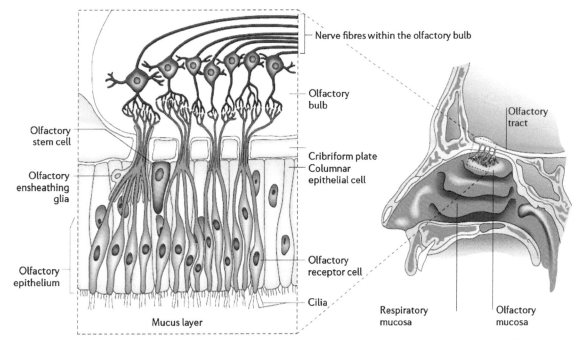

FIG. 1.6 Olfactory concussion: posttraumatic symptoms arising from damage to the olfactory nerves, bulbs, or tracts such as diminished or exaggerated smell. (Reprinted with permission from Thuret S, Moon LDF, Gage FH. Therapeutic interventions after spinal cord injury. *Nature Reviews. Neuroscience.* 2006;7:628–643.)

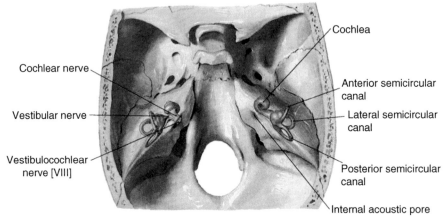

FIG. 1.7 Vestibular and auditory concussion. Vestibular concussion: posttraumatic symptoms arising from dysfunction of the semicircular canals, such as dizziness, balance problems, and lightheadedness. Auditory concussion: posttraumatic symptoms arising from cochlear dysfunction such as hyperacousis or hypoacousis, sensitivity to noise. (From Paulsen F. Ear. In: *Sobotta Atlas of Human Anatomy*. 15th ed. Munich: Elsevier, Fig. 10.39.)

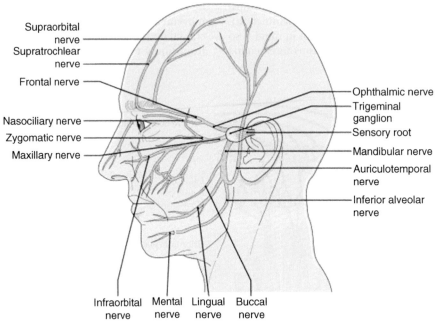

FIG. 1.8 Trigeminal concussion: posttraumatic symptoms arising from stimulation or depression of the branches of the trigeminal nerve, such as headache, facial pain, or numbness. (From Grant GA, Loeser JD. Trigeminal Neuralgia. In: Ellenbogen, Richard G, ed. *Principles of Neurological Surgery*. 3rd ed. Philadelphia: Elsevier; 2012, Fig. 48.1.)

of a retinal concussion causing alterations of retinal function, leading to diminished, dim, or fuzzy vision, as well as photophobia or visual aberrations. One can have a trigeminal concussion that may give rise to different types of facial pain and numbness (Fig. 1.8).

The first three cervical nerve roots are involved with a type of pain that can produce a cervicogenic headache, and these roots do communicate with the trigeminal nerve through the brain stem in addition to peripheral branches going up the back of the head

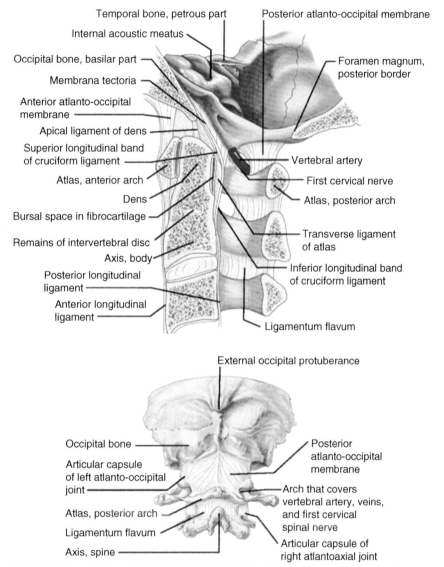

FIG. 1.9 Cervical concussion: posttraumatic symptoms arising from the nerves, muscles, joints, ligaments, or blood vessels in the neck such as neck pain, numbness or pain in the posterior portion of the head, and lightheadedness. (From Standring S, ed. *Gray's Anatomy*. 40th ed. Edinburgh: Elsevier Churchill Livingstone; 2009:733.)

as the greater and lesser occipital nerves. We can also have symptoms that can arise from the nerves, muscles, and joints in our cervical spine itself (Fig. 1.9). We can also have what we think of as spinal concussion symptoms arising from the upper spinal cord itself, such as paralysis, numbness, and weakness (Fig. 1.10). Lastly, we can have psychological concussion, posttraumatic cognitive and psychological symptoms arising from the influence of mechanical energy on one's overall psychological state. This topic is a complex issue, but suffice it to say that the brain enters a state of being stressed with mechanical forces that lead to challenges such as poor attention, depression, anxiety, migraine, and other symptoms. It is likely that the magnitude and expression of these symptoms will depend not only on the magnitude of the mechanical input, but also on the psychological and personality factors.

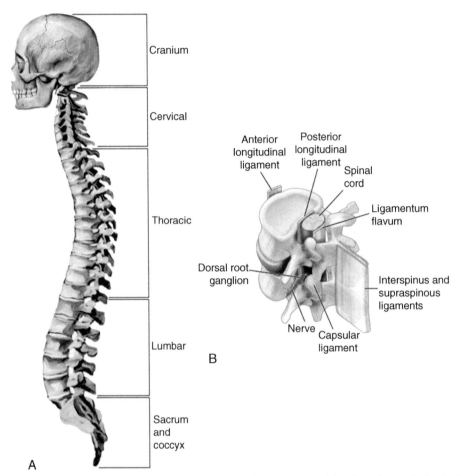

FIG. 1.10 Spinal cord (**A** and **B**) concussion: posttraumatic symptoms arising from the cervical spinal cord such as tingling, numbness, and weakness. (From Jaumard NV, Syre PP, Welch WC, Winkelstein BA. Head and Spine Anatomy and Biomechanics. In: Mark Miller, ed. *DeLee & Drez's Orthopaedic Sports Medicine*. 4th ed. Philadelphia: Elsevier; 2015, Fig. 121.1.)

Current Definitions of Concussion

So concussion today is really defined by mechanically induced symptoms, and the symptoms no longer exclusively involve the brain, but also other structures in the head and neck. When we look at our symptom checklist that many of us use, we look at the number of symptoms and their severity, and that information along with our cognitive, eye tracking, and balance assessments are the four main pillars of concussion assessment today (Fig. 1.11). Note that many of the symptoms on the checklist are not cerebral symptoms; they are from the other head and neck structures that we described.

So are we seeing more concussions today? I think the answer is "yes," and it's "yes" because people are

bigger, stronger, and faster and the forces involved are greater than ever before. I also agree with all of you that we are identifying them better today—we are still missing a significant percentage but certainly fewer than we did in the past. Yet another reason that we are seeing more concussions today is because we liberalized the definition of concussion and made it symptom based. The forces needed to impart some of those symptoms are not as great as the forces that are needed to cause loss of consciousness, the definition of concussion way back in the day.

I have just returned from Berlin and the Fifth International Concussion Conference that was held last week, where 12 questions were discussed in great detail

ROBERT C. CANTU, MA, MD, FACS,FAANS, FICS, FACSM
TODAY'S CONCUSSION SIGNS/SYMPTOMS CHECKLIST

Patient Name:_____   Date:_____

Today's Date / Date of Concussion	None	Mild	Moderate	Severe				Today's Date / Date of Concussion	None	Mild	Moderate	Severe			
	0	1	2	3	4	5	6		0	1	2	3	4	5	6
Balance Issues								Nausea/Vomiting							
Confusion								Neck Pain							
Difficulty Concentrating								Nervous/Anxious							
Difficulty Remembering								Numbness/Tingling							
Dizziness								Ringing in the Ears							
Don't Feel Right/Dinged/Bell Rung								Sadness							
Drowsy								Sensitivity to Light							
Fatigue/Low Energy								Sensitivity to Noise							
Feeling In A Fog								Sleeping Less than Usual							
Feeling More Emotional								Sleeping More than Usual							
Feeling Slowed Down								Trouble Falling Asleep							
Headache/Head Pressure								Visual Problems/Blurred Vision							
Irritability															
Loss of Consciousness	No Loc	<15 sec	15-30 sec	30-45 sec	45-60 sec	>60 sec									

The athlete should score themselves on the above symptoms based on how they feel today. (i.e. 0 = not pre:
1-2 = mild, 3-4 = moderate, 5-6 = severe).

©Copyright – No reproductions without permission
For Dr. Cantu's Use Only:

Symptom Load _____/26   Symptom Score_____/156   Concussion Grade_____

FIG. 1.11 Today's concussion signs and symptoms checklist, by Robert C. Cantu, MA, MD, FACS, FAANS, FICS, FACSM. (Figure courtesy of Dr. Cantu. ©Copyright—no reproductions without written permission from Dr. Cantu.)

that will be tackled in the new consensus document and will be the subject of individual scientific endeavors. The first question is, "What is the definition of concussion?" The group decided that "concussion is a traumatic brain injury and is defined as a complex pathophysiological process affecting the brain, induced by biomechanical forces." I am very pleased that the group has finally moved to calling concussion a "traumatic brain injury"—not a "*mild* traumatic brain injury." I realize where the "mild" came from, but when someone has symptoms that are prolonged, and someone has issues that have totally changed their life, it is inappropriate to call that a "mild" brain injury just because you can't see macroscopic trauma on a brain imaging study, especially when we are now seeing from Dr. McKee and others the microscopic injury of concussion that may cause a number of structural issues in the brain (Chapter 2).

CHRONIC TRAUMATIC ENCEPHALOPATHY IN ATHLETES

My involvement in the history of CTE started in 1995 when we wrote a book, *Boxing and Medicine* (Fig. 1.12).[6] There were a number of chapters and one was on traumatic brain injury in boxers and we covered in some detail the CTE issue. I am sure all of you have heard of, if you haven't seen it yourself, the movie *Concussion*, about Bennet Omalu's life and discoveries. It was not quite true that he found a disease that nobody had ever seen before, because he didn't discover CTE and he did not name chronic traumatic encephalopathy, but we should give him tremendous credit for having discovered the first case of it in a National Football League (NFL) player, Mike Webster, and subsequent players. So he saw CTE in an NFL player and also wrote it up in the journal *Neurosurgery* (Fig. 1.13).[7]

CTE in Boxers

However, the person who first described the clinical syndrome of CTE was Harrison Martland back in 1928[8] (Fig. 1.14). He was a coroner in New Jersey and had an interest in boxers. He was at ringside a lot, and he described the clinical pattern of cognitive, behavioral, and mood issues that these boxers manifested. He called it "punch drunk" syndrome. He also had the insight to realize—because of his personal involvement being there ringside—it was the boxer who had tremendous exposure with the greatest number of fights who was most likely to show this clinical triad. If a boxer was

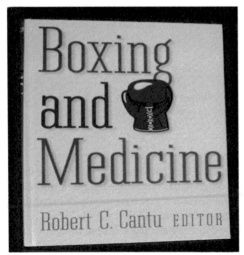

FIG. 1.12 Boxing and medicine. Robert C. Cantu, editor. Published 1995 by Human Kinetics Publishers. (Figure courtesy of Dr. Cantu.)

showing this syndrome but didn't have a large number of fights, then he would have fought for a long period of time, or be the type of boxer who was primarily a slugger, who took a lot of blows to give one. Martland recognized these issues back in 1928.

I also think that it's an interesting side note that in his paper that he published in the *Journal of the American Medical Association* in 1928 there are a couple of paragraphs about Gene Tunney, who held the heavyweight boxing title from 1926 to 1928. In preparation for a fight, Tunney was knocked down during a sparring session. He got up and finished the sparring session but was amnestic as he had no memory of the sparring session in which he knocked out his sparring partner. This happened on a Friday and he had no memory of Saturday or Sunday either. Tunney realized, because he had good common sense, "I got hit in the head and lost the weekend." So he used his mind and decided he was going to retire from boxing if he won his next match. He did win, and he retired from boxing and he went on to have a very successful business career and long life, dying at age 81.

Corsellis first described the pathology of CTE in 15 ex-boxers in terms of the morphology. He stressed the cavum septum and the atrophy, including the mammillary bodies and fornix, the cerebellar tonsillar scarring, pallor of the substantia nigra, and the neurofibrillary tangles.[9] It remained for Dr. McKee to really define exactly where those neurofibrillary tangles needed to be for the hallmark diagnosis of CTE (Chapter 2).

In terms of who actually first used the words "chronic traumatic encephalopathy," we have Martland describing the symptoms under the term "punch drunk," and we had others talking about it as "dementia pugilistica," "psychopathic deterioration of the pugilist," and then we had Macdonald Critchley, first in a book chapter to Vincent, a French neurosurgeon, and then in the *British Medical Journal*, describing what the boxers were experiencing as "chronic progressive traumatic encephalopathy" and "chronic traumatic encephalopathy."[10]

Early Recognition in Football Players

All right, so in 1928 we had the clinical syndrome identified and described by Martland. Look what was in newspapers in the 1930s (Fig. 1.15). We recently discovered case reports of "punch-drunk" football players, "stumble-backs" in the early literature. This newspaper article was taken from the *Columbia Daily Spectator* in 1937: "Punch-drunk football stars" and "stumble-backs—does football make players stupid?" So we really had some clinical descriptions of CTE

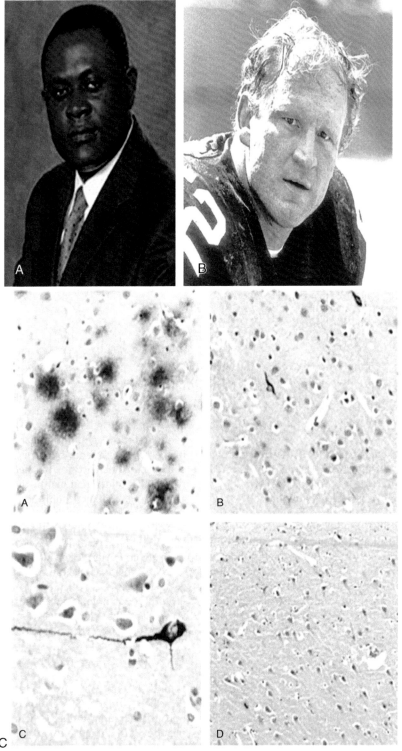

FIG. 1.13 (A) Bennet Omalu, (B) Mike Webster, and (C) the first report of chronic traumatic encephalopathy in a football player. (From Omalu BI, DeKosky ST, Minster RL, Kamboh MI, Hamilton RL, Wecht CH. Chronic traumatic encephalopathy in a National Football League player. *Neurosurgery*. July 2005; 57(1):128–134; Discussion 128–134. PMID: 15987548.)

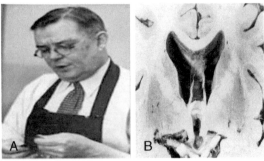

FIG. 1.14 **(A)** In 1928 Harrison Martland, a coroner in New Jersey, identifies the clinical pattern of cognitive and behavioral issues that he called "punch drunk syndrome," which would be subsequently identified as dementia pugilistica and ultimately chronic traumatic encephalopathy (CTE). **(B)** In 1973, Corsellis and colleagues first describe the pathology in 15 ex-boxers. Gross pathology image showing a cavum septum, a common feature in CTE. ((A) Image courtesy of Dr. Cantu. (B) From Corsellis JA, Bruton CJ, Freeman-Browne D. The aftermath of boxing. *Psychological Medicine*. August 1973;3(3):270–303. PMID: 4729191.)

in football players a long time ago, but it dropped out of the public discussion and out of the public awareness.

The Boston University Team Working to Understand CTE

At BU this is the team I have had the tremendous pleasure to be associated with (Fig. 1.16). Formed in 2008, the Center for the Study of CTE includes Mr. Christopher Nowinski, the brain chaser, the one who obtains the brains for Dr. McKee to study. Dr. Stern is involved with longitudinal studies looking to define the clinical syndrome more precisely, and to find biomarkers to detect CTE in living individuals (Chapter 3). More recently, Dr. Goldstein has come on the scene to understand the mechanism of CTE pathology (Chapter 5). The center has subsequently been combined with the BU Alzheimer's Disease Center, and we are now a team with Dr. Neil Kowall, its director.

When Dr. McKee published her original research paper in 2009 describing additional cases of CTE and reviewing the 45 cases in the world literature, it was the most comprehensive review of CTE at that time. Just a few years later she added an additional 68 cases of CTE to the world literature, and she ultimately gave us the neuropathological diagnostic criteria of CTE, as well as a pathological CTE severity scale, and I will let her describe all of that, and what she has found in various groups of athletes.

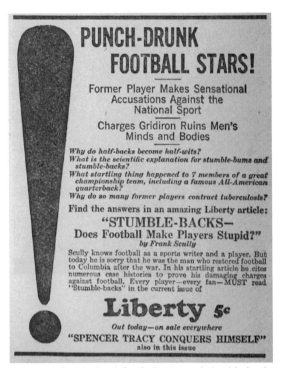

FIG. 1.15 Punch-drunk football stars and stumble-backs: does football make players stupid? (Figure from *Columbia Daily Spectator*, vol. LXI, Number 6; September 29, 1937.)

One of the biggest things that has happened in CTE in the last 50 years has been Dr. McKee's convening a consensus conference for the neuropathological criteria for CTE under National Institutes of Health (NIH) sanctioning, and then publishing the findings of that conference. So today we have a footprint for what CTE is pathologically, and we are no longer having people questioning whether CTE is really a form of Alzheimer's or an atypical neurodegeneration mixed with something else. We know that CTE can coexist with other neurodegenerative diseases (Chapter 8), but CTE has a specific footprint of pathology at the base of sulci around blood vessels, and that perivascular distribution of pathology must be there if you're going to call it CTE.

CTE Has Been Found in Many Contact Sports

I think all of you know that CTE has now been described virtually in every type of athlete that sustains brain trauma. Some of the more recent additions include BMX biking and mixed martial arts, which are not a surprise. One recent study by Bieniek et al.[11] analyzed neurodegenerative disorders in their brain bank using the NIH consensus criteria that Dr. McKee's group developed. When they looked at the group that

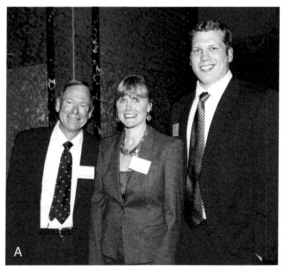

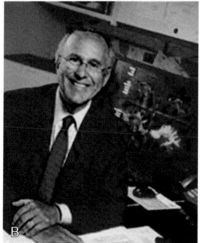

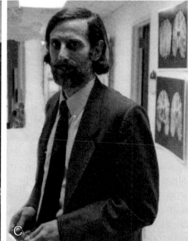

FIG. 1.16 Leaders of the Boston University chronic traumatic encephalopathy research team. **(A)** (left to right) Robert Cantu, Ann McKee, Christopher Nowinski. **(B)** Robert Stern. **(C)** Lee Goldstein. (Images courtesy of Dr. Cantu.)

had contact sport exposure, they found CTE in 32%, in contrast to 0% in the group without contact.

Unforgotten: The Paul Pender Story

In September 2016 I was filling in for Dr. McKee, who is the star of a motion picture called *Unforgotten: The Paul Pender Story*, and I was asked to be on a panel to discuss CTE with sports writers, scientists, and one boxer (Fig. 1.17). Paul Pender was a Brookline student who started boxing in high school and embarked on a professional career that took him to age 30 when he defeated Sugar Ray Robinson at the Boston Garden, so he held a portion of the middleweight title at that

time. He was thought of as a boxer puncher. He didn't take a lot of trauma and he had a broken hand four times and he also needed surgery, so he had his career interrupted. He didn't have quite as many exposures as you would have thought for someone who fought from his teenage years to age 33 because there were periods in-between when he couldn't fight. By the time when he was in his 50s he had to be taken care of by his wife, and in his later 50s he was institutionalized at the Bedford Veterans Affairs Hospital where Dr. McKee was working at the time, and she will tell you what she ultimately found when she came to examine his brain (Chapter 2).

DAY FOUR
SUNDAY, SEPTEMBER 25

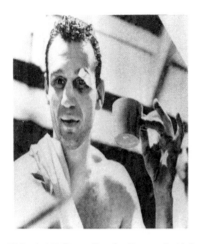

UNFORGOTTEN: THE PAUL PENDER STORY
5:00PM (64 M) - AMC BOSTON COMMON

Q&A Felice Leeds, Paul Pender, Jr., Mike Silver, Richard Johnson, Tony DeMarco and Robert Cantu, world-renowned CTE expert, B.U.

The extraordinary story of Boston's own Golden Age boxer - from his struggles overcoming physical adversity to his against-the-odds victory over Sugar Ray Robinson to become World Champion. Later in life he suffers from the debilitating brain disease CTE, and his brain study starts a movement that transforms the future of sports.

DIRECTOR: Felice Leeds PRODUCER: Bennett Leeds NARRATOR: Mary Babbitt STARRING: Dr. Ann McKee, Bud Collins, Tony DeMarco and former Governor Michael Dukakis

FIG. 1.17 Promotion for the movie *Unforgotten: The Paul Pender Story.* (Figure courtesy of Dr. Cantu.)

With me that night on the discussion panel was Tony DeMarco (Fig. 1.18). Tony was a welterweight champion at the same time Paul Pender was fighting as a middleweight. Tony DeMarco was an individual who was thought of as a slugger more than a boxer puncher. He had a lengthy career and, despite this fact, there he was, a couple of chairs away from me that night with his wife. I can't attest to whether he had subtle issues going on, but he was certainly pleasant to chat with.

THE FUTURE OF CONCUSSION AND CTE IN ATHLETES
Important Questions to Be Answered About CTE

We certainly still have a number of questions that need to be answered in this area. Today we are not knowledgeable about the incidence or prevalence of CTE, or what exposure is needed to get CTE. The exact exposure is probably going to vary greatly between different people, as CTE has been seen in football players as young as those in high school. We don't yet know the risk factors that make you more or less likely to develop CTE. Although the pathological criteria have been defined, and great strides have been made toward defining the clinical syndrome of CTE, there is more work to be done in recognizing the disease clinically and in understanding its pathophysiology.

Increasing Recognition of CTE

One of the biggest changes that we have been able to see happen with the International Concussion Consensus group has been in relation to CTE. Some of their key questions in the conference last week in Berlin included:

- "What is the current state of the scientific evidence about the prevalence, risk factors, and causation of possible long-term sequelae like CTE and other neurodegenerative diseases, with respect to sports concussion?"
- "What are the definition, clinical features, and underlying pathophysiology (if any) of 'sub-concussive blows' and how can they be measured and monitored?"
- "What have we learned from the retired athlete population?"

After many years of denial, in March 2016 the NFL admitted the link between CTE and exposure to head hits in football. I think this admission came about because they were present when Dr. McKee presented her quite compelling material in a congressional hearing. The NFL was one of the first major sporting bodies to make this statement, following the World Rugby Association. We are still waiting for other major international sporting groups to acknowledge the link, groups like the International Olympic Committee, Fédération Internationale de Football Association (FIFA), the International Equestrian Federation, and the National Hockey League (NHL).

With that, I thank you very much.

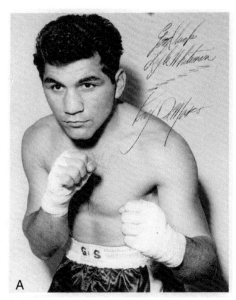
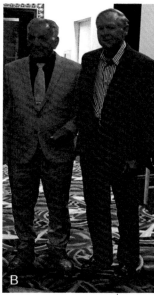

FIG. 1.18 Tony DeMarco **(A)** in 2016, left, with Dr. Cantu, right **(B)**. (Image courtesy of Dr. Cantu.)

DISCLOSURES

Senior advisor, NFL Head, Neck and Spine Committee. Vice President, National Operating Committee on Standards for Athletic Equipment (NOCSAE), and Chair, Scientific Advisory Committee. Cofounder, Concussion Legacy Foundation. Royalties from Houghton Mifflin Harcourt. Legal Expert Opinion.

REFERENCES

1. Cantu RC. Guidelines for return to contact sports after a cerebral concussion. *The Physician and Sportsmedicine*. October 1986;14(10):75–83. http://dx.doi.org/10.1080/0091 3847.1986.11709197. PMID: 27432133.
2. Cantu RC. Posttraumatic retrograde and anterograde amnesia: pathophysiology and implications in grading and safe return to play. *Journal of Athletic Training*. September 2001;36(3):244–248. PMID: 12937491.
3. McCrory P, Meeuwisse WH, Aubry M, et al. Consensus statement on concussion in sport: the 4th International Conference on Concussion in Sport held in Zurich, November 2012. *British Journal of Sports Medicine*. April 2013;47(5):250–258. http://dx.doi.org/10.1136/bjsports-2013-092313. PMID: 23479479.
4. Gennarelli TA. The centripetal theory of concussion (CTC) revisited after 40 years and a proposed new symptomcentric concept of the concussions, IRCOBI, IRC-15-02, 2015, Lyon, France. pp VIII-XIII. http://www.ircobi.org/wordpress/downloads/irc15/pdf_files/02.pdf[ircobi.org].
5. Gennarelli TA. What do we know about angular head motions. In IRCOBI-NOCSAE-Snell-PDB, TBI Workshop, Lyon, France, 2015. http://www.ircobi.org/downloads/ircobi-head-workshop-2015.pdf[ircobi.org].
6. Cantu RC, ed. *Boxing and Medicine*. Human Kinetics Publishers; March 1995. ISBN-10: 0873227972 ISBN-13: 978–0873227971.
7. Omalu BI, DeKosky ST, Minster RL, Kamboh MI, Hamilton RL, Wecht CH. Chronic traumatic encephalopathy in a National Football League player. *Neurosurgery*. July 2005;57(1):128–134. Discussion 128–134. PMID: 15987548.
8. Martland HS. Punch drunk. *JAMA*. 1928;91(15):1103–1107. http://dx.doi.org/10.1001/jama.1928.02700150029009.
9. Corsellis JA, Bruton CJ, Freeman-Browne D. The aftermath of boxing. *Psychological Medicine*. August 1973;3(3):270–303. PMID: 4729191.
10. Critchley M. Medical aspects of boxing, particularly from a neurological standpoint. *British Medical Journal*. February 16, 1957:357–362.
11. Bieniek KF, Ross OA, Cormier KA, et al. Chronic traumatic encephalopathy pathology in a neurodegenerative disorders brain bank. *Acta Neuropathologica*. 2015;130(6):877–889.

FURTHER READING

1. Montenigro PH, Corp DT, Stein TD, Cantu RC, Stern RA. Chronic traumatic encephalopathy: historical origins and current perspective. *Annual Review of Clinical Psychology*. 2015;11:309–330. http://dx.doi.org/10.1146/annurev-clinpsy-032814-112814. PMID: 25581233.
2. Ommaya AK, Gennarelli TA. Cerebral concussion and traumatic unconsciousness. Correlation of experimental and clinical observations of blunt head injuries. *Brain*. December 1974;97(4):633–654. PMID: 4215541.
3. Shaw N. Neurophysiology of concussion: theoretical perspectives. In: Slobounov SM, Sebastianelli WJ, eds. *Foundations of Sport-Related Brain Injuries*. 2006th ed. Springer; May 3, 2006. ISBN-10: 0387325646 ISBN-13: 978–0387325644.

CHAPTER 2

Pathology of Chronic Traumatic Encephalopathy

ANN C. MCKEE • THOR D. STEIN • BERTRAND R. HUBER • VICTOR E. ALVAREZ

INTRODUCTION

Good morning. First, let me say that the work I am going to present is really a team effort. We wouldn't be anywhere without an incredible team. I have a wonderful group of neuropathologists who I work with: Dr. Thor Stein, Dr. Russ Huber, and Dr. Victor Alvarez, who all contribute every day to this work. But it's the research assistants, the graduate students, the post docs, and the doctoral students that commit themselves 24 h a day to this effort that make it all happen. They get paid very little but they are so committed—they do the work because of all the families of the donors to our center. (Turning to the families) It's such a privilege to have you here. I am so honored by the families being here. This work is about you and we never forget that. This work is about people, the loved ones you lost, and we want to tell their stories because they can't.

So I am going to talk about chronic traumatic encephalopathy (CTE) and where we have come in the last 8 years. It is true that the neuropathology has been not only important but actually was the key to defining this disease. Eventually, we will have clinical criteria to define CTE, but right now, we know this is a real disease because it has a defining pathology. The pathology of CTE is unique—it's not the pathology of Alzheimer's disease or aging or anything else that you might hear from others. This is an actual, specific disease that can be easily diagnosed microscopically—and it is not rare. We know it's not rare because we have received more than 250 instances of this disease over the past 8 years. So unless we are magicians (and I know we are not), this disease is much more common than most people appreciate. CTE is not rare, CTE is easily diagnosed if you look for it, and CTE is a consequence of repetitive head trauma.

CTE IS COMMON IN CONTACT SPORT ATHLETES

It all started with John Grimsley and Tom McHale, the first brain donors to our center. John and Tom were former football players for the National Football League (NFL), and they both played for 9 years. They both retired in their early 30s. And in their early 40s, they both developed symptoms—subtle behavioral symptoms. Their wives and families didn't know exactly what to make of their behavior changes, but they knew something was different. John and Tom both died at the age of 45 from accidental causes, and both their families donated their brains to the center, which was really the beginning of the CTE center. What we found in those brains, in those 45-year-olds, was an extraordinary neurodegenerative disease called CTE. I had seen it one time before in the world champion boxer Paul Pender, who died at the age of 73 years, and it knocked me out of my socks. In 25 years of looking at brains I had never seen a brain like Paul Pender's (Fig. 2.1). I thought it was something extraordinary, and I tried to find similar cases in our brain bank. I couldn't. It was 5 years later when we got the cases of Tom and John that I saw this same disease in the brains of two 45-year-olds. I've been working on neurodegenerative diseases for my entire life, and I was comfortable with people getting older and sick and getting Alzheimer's or Parkinson's disease, but I had never in my life seen a neurodegenerative disease like CTE in a person only 45 years old.

So this was something that was truly extraordinary, and that is why Dr. Robert Stern, Dr. Robert Cantu, Chris Nowinski, and I put together what we call the Veterans Affairs-Boston University-Concussion Legacy Foundation (VA-BU-CLF) brain bank to try and to investigate the long-term consequences of mild traumatic brain injury. We have 365 brain donors at this

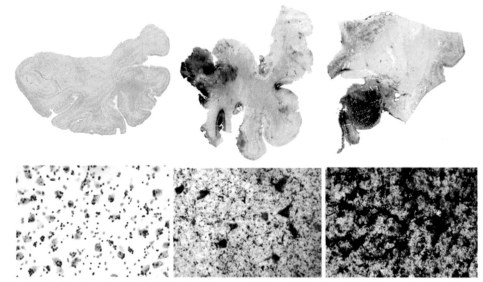

FIG. 2.1 Brain autopsies of John Grimsley, 45-year-old former NFL player (middle), and Paul Pender, 73-year-old former boxer (right), compared with a control subject (left). *Brown staining* represents tau pathology. (Figure courtesy of Dr. McKee.)

point—truly extraordinary—and we are getting brains at a rate of about seven per month. That is extraordinary, and it's because of the commitment of families. Most of these brains are coming in because families are reaching out to us.

By now, we have looked at a lot of brains from football players. Most of our cases, 260, have come from football players (Table 2.1). We also get brains from military veterans, and we are trying to increase the numbers of brain we receive from veterans. We receive brains from other athletes as well, including wrestlers, hockey players, boxers, soccer players, and we've seen a lot of CTE. The fact that families are sending us these brains and we are finding CTE in them is another clue that this cannot be rare. Either the families are really good at diagnosing this disease in life, or this disease is much more common than was previously believed.

We find CTE in 72% of brain donors, 222 positive for CTE out of 308 evaluated (Table 2.2). That percentage is extraordinarily high. Our criterion for getting into the brain bank is exposure to mild head trauma over a long time. And it turns out a lot of these guys have CTE.

PATHOLOGIC FEATURES OF CTE

What are the diagnostic features of CTE? Over the years we've really honed it down to two essential

TABLE 2.1
Veterans Affairs-Boston University-Concussion Legacy Foundation Brain Donors

Exposure	Number of Brain Donors
Boxing	16
American football	260
Ice hockey	18
Professional wrestling	6
Rugby	7
Military veterans*	27 (*also 65 veteran-athletes counted under athletes)
Soccer	5
Other sport: amateur wrestling, baseball, bull riding, lacrosse, martial arts, water polo	12
Other: physical abuse, poorly controlled epilepsy, head banging, law enforcement	14
Total	365

TABLE 2.2
CTE Diagnoses in the Veterans Affairs-Boston University-Concussion Legacy Foundation Brain Bank

Exposure	Number of Brain Donors With CTE	Number of Brain Donors Evaluated
Boxing	14	16
American football	177	214
Ice hockey	9	16
Professional wrestling	2	4
Rugby	3	6
Military veterans*	10 (*51 veteran-athletes)	24 (*60 veteran-athletes)
Soccer	3	5
Other sport: amateur wrestling, baseball, bull riding, lacrosse, martial arts, water polo	3	12
Other: Physical abuse, poorly controlled epilepsy, head banging	1	11
Total	222	308

features. First, there is the pathology around blood vessels. There is no other neurodegenerative disease that has pathology like this in Fig. 2.2A. There is no other disease in which abnormal tau protein is deposited around blood vessels. This distribution is truly remarkable. It defines the disease. The tau is not just in neurons as neurofibrillary tangles or in neurites, it is also in astrocytes. So abnormal tau is in cells surrounding blood vessels, and that is a defining feature of the CTE. Second, the tau around blood vessels occurs in the crevices of the brain—in the depths of the sulci—usually in the frontal cortex and also in the temporal cortex (Fig. 2.2B).

The Physics of Brain Injury Determines the Location of Pathology

Why is the tau pathology in those regions? Because of the physics of brain injury. When individuals are subjected to the acceleration, deceleration, and rotation injuries that happen in every play on the football field, the shearing forces are the greatest at the bottom of the crevices (Fig. 2.3). We all know this—it's like when you open a bag of potato chips, it opens at the crevices of the crenulations. And we know it's greatest along the blood vessels. You have relatively stiff blood vessels inside a gelatinous brain and when you start shaking it up and jarring it, you get damage distributed around those stiff blood vessels, and that's why we see the tau there, because that is where the damage is the greatest. You'll hear more about this from Dr. Lee Goldstein (Chapter 5).

Consensus Criteria Established

For a long time it seemed like I had to fight the world to prove CTE was a real disease. I have never in my life had an experience like this where people were saying I was making up a disease or confusing it with some other disease, like Alzheimer's disease. I knew that we could never begin to work toward what was important—developing treatments—unless we could convince people that CTE was a real disease. So after about 5 years the National Institute of Neurologic Disorders and Stroke supported a grant that brought together a panel of expert neuropathologists from many academic institutions (Fig. 2.4). My colleague, Dr. Thor Stein, was one of them. We also had experts from places like Seattle, Mayo Clinic, Columbia, Washington University, and these premier neuropathologists looked at 700 slides that I gave them. Note that these were undesignated slides—there were no labels to indicate what the case was or what type of person—a football player, a boxer, or an elderly female—it came from. Those 700 slides represented 25 cases, identically stained, labeled, and there was no other information provided to the neuropathologists who were analyzing them. I asked them, based on the criteria we proposed, could they tell which of these cases are CTE? This was a really difficult test because they had to distinguish CTE from other diseases which also had abnormal tau pathology such as corticobasal degeneration, progressive supranuclear palsy, and even Parkinsonism-dementia complex of Guam—which, I'd like to add, most of us had never

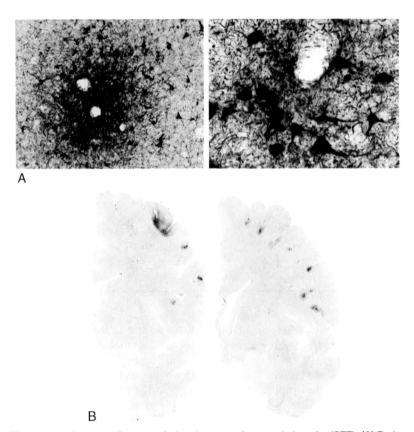

A

B

FIG. 2.2 The primary diagnostic features of chronic traumatic encephalopathy (CTE). **(A)** Perivascular p-tau lesion. **(B)** Pathology distributed at the depths of the cortical sulci. (With permission from McKee AC, et al. The spectrum of disease in chronic traumatic encephalopathy. *Brain*. January 2013;136(Pt 1):43–64. http://dx.doi.org/10.1093/brain/aws307. Erratum in: *Brain*. October 2013;136(Pt 10):e255.)

even seen a case of. So this was a difficult task. It took each neuropathologist about 100 h, and at the end of the day, it turned out that there was tremendous agreement. The neuropathologists agreed that there was pathognomonic lesion of CTE—a lesion that defines this disease—and that CTE was distinct from all other neurodegenerations. They agreed that CTE was a very unique tauopathy. The lesion that they all agreed was pathognomonic was the perivascular accumulation of tau at the depths of the sulci (Fig. 2.5).[1] They also said that in their experience it has resulted from repeated trauma. So what this panel determined last year is that CTE is a disease, a distinct disease—it is not Alzheimer's and not aging. There was agreement that the diagnosis of CTE can be definitive by examination of brain tissue, and that it's only after trauma that we see it. This was a huge step forward.

Consensus Criteria Independently Verified

Then Kevin Bieniek, a young investigator at the Mayo Clinic, looked through 1700 autopsy male brains—a huge amount of work—for changes of CTE. He found CTE in 21 brains, and, lo and behold, all 21 were contact sports athletes. In fact, when he looked at all the cases, about one-third of the contact sports athletes in the brain bank had changes of CTE.[2] What these results indicate is that CTE is more common than most people realize—if you look for it, you can find it, and it is associated with contact sports. Also important is that he didn't see CTE in controls, in people without brain trauma. This is another key point. Lastly, when he looked at 33 brains with a history of a single traumatic brain injury, none of these cases had CTE. So, we have an independent neuropathologist at another medical center who has verified our main findings using their brain bank.

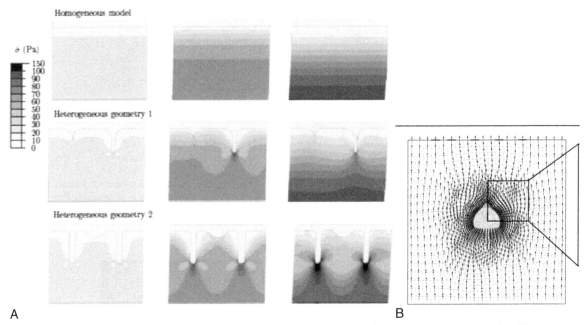

A   B

FIG. 2.3 The bottom of the sulci and perivascular areas are regions of physical stress concentration. **(A)** Strain fields as a result of different geometries. Heterogeneous geometries 1 and 2 are closest to the human brain with sulci. **(B)** Strain field around a rigid object, as could occur around a blood vessel. ((A) With permission from Cloots, et al. *Annals of Biomedical Engineering*, vol. 36, No. 7, July 2008. (B) With permission from Cloots, et al. *The Journal of the Mechanical Behavior of Biomedical Materials*. 2012:41–52.)

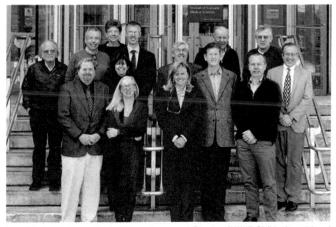

FIG. 2.4 National Institute of Neurologic Disorders and Stroke (NINDS)/National Institute of Biomedical Imaging and Bioengineering (NIBIB) Consensus meeting to evaluate pathological criteria for the diagnosis of CTE. Held February 25 to 26, 2015; the consensus members included: Nigel Cairns, PhD; Rebecca Folkerth, MD; Wayne Gordon PhD; C. Dirk Keene, MD; Irene Litvan, PhD; Ann McKee, MD; Daniel Perl, MD; Thor Stein MD, PhD; William Stewart, MD; Jean Paul Vonsattel, MD; Dennis Dickson, MD; Patrick Bellgowan, MD; Debra Babcock, PhD; Walter Koroschetz, MD. For more information see http://www.ninds.nih.gov/research/tbi/ReportFirstNIHConsensusConference.htm. (Figure courtesy of Dr. McKee.)

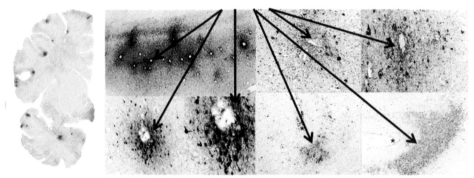

FIG. 2.5 The pathognomonic lesion of CTE. "In CTE, the Tau Lesion Considered pathognomonic was an Abnormal Perivascular Accumulation of Tau in Neurons, Astrocytes, and Cell Processes in an Irregular Pattern at the Depths of the Cortical Sulci." Quote From the Consensus Conference, http://www.ninds.nih.gov/research/tbi/ReportFirstNIHConsensusConference.htm. (Figure courtesy of Dr. McKee.)

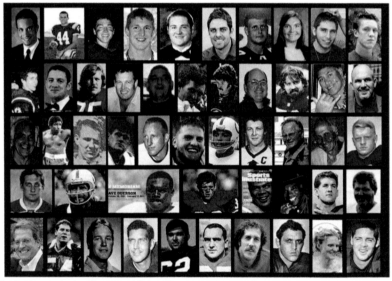

FIG. 2.6 Brain donors in the Veterans Affairs-Boston University-Concussion Legacy Foundation (VA-BU-CLF) brain bank, all but four with pathologic diagnoses of CTE. (Figure courtesy of Dr. McKee.)

CTE Spreads Through the Brain Even After the Trauma Has Stopped

So this is a disease about people. A lot of these loved ones you can see in Fig. 2.6 have family members here at the conference. I want to talk about their cases and what we see in their brains. The youngest members in our brain bank can be seen in the top row, with older members in lower rows. They played football, hockey, and wrestling. They represent people who took their own life, people who died in accidents, and also people who led long lives but at the end developed severe disease.

So what do you see in their brains? In Fig. 2.7, you can see the brains of individuals in the top row with the least amount of disease—the youngest individuals showing just one or two perivascular CTE lesions. When the disease gets more severe you see more perivascular lesions involving more of the brain, and finally in the middle and bottom rows it starts to spread. It spreads to involve other parts of the brain. And that is a key point. The individuals in these lower levels stopped playing football and other sports long before they died, but the disease progressed and started involving other parts of the

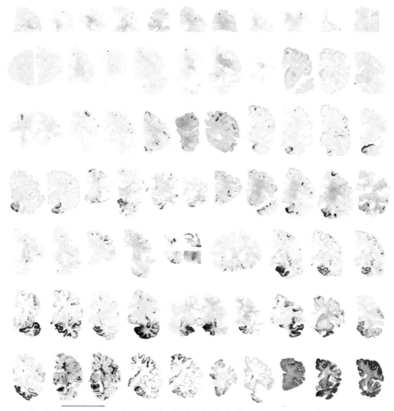

FIG. 2.7 The pathologic spectrum of CTE. The individuals in the top rows are the youngest members in the brain bank with the least amount of disease, just one or two perivascular lesions. the disease is more severe in the middle rows, involving more of the brain, and in the bottom rows it has spread to involve many parts of the brain. (With permission from McKee AC, et al. The spectrum of disease in chronic traumatic encephalopathy. *Brain*. January 2013;136(Pt 1):43–64. http://dx.doi.org/10.1093/brain/aws307. Erratum in: *Brain*. October 2013;136(Pt 10):e255.)

brain. This is another key point. There is a spreading phenomenon, and we need to understand why this disease is progressive in the absence of ongoing trauma.

Stages of CTE

We divided CTE into four stages of pathology (Fig. 2.8). Stage I involves just a few lesions and is usually asymptomatic. Stage II has more lesions scattered throughout the brain, and is still often asymptomatic. Stage III is where the disease starts to involve the medial temporal lobe, including the parts of the brain that control memory and learning. Stage IV is when it's throughout the brain.

We found in our cases that the staging of the pathology significantly correlated with the age of death, meaning the older individuals had more severe,

higher stages of CTE. Disease stage also correlated with years of playing football—an important concept. The longer you play football, the greater is the severity of your CTE.

Young Individuals With CTE

Erik Pelly, who was 18 when he died, was our second case of CTE (Fig. 2.9). I was expecting a pristine brain. An 18-year-old's brain is still modeling and still laying down white matter tracks. It's still pruning synapses. It should be pristine. Instead, in his brain I could see several lesions. They were apparent to the naked eye, and when we looked under the microscope we could see that there were perivascular lesions around small blood vessels. That finding is very abnormal. I had never seen an 18-year-old with focal neurodegeneration of this magnitude.

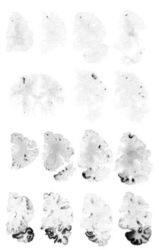

FIG. 2.8 Stages of tau pathology in CTE. CTE stage is significantly correlated with age at death and duration of exposure to football. First row: stage I, mean age 28.3±13 years. Second row: stage II, mean age 44.3±16 years. Third row: stage III, mean age 56.0±14 years. Fourth row: stage IV, mean age 77.4±12 years. (With permission from McKee AC, et al. The spectrum of disease in chronic traumatic encephalopathy. *Brain*. January 2013;136(Pt 1):43–64. http://dx.doi.org/10.1093/brain/aws307. Erratum in: *Brain*. 2013. October 2013;136(Pt 10):e255.)

We have also seen CTE in college players. This is Michael Keck, who died at the age of 25 (Fig. 2.10). He played 3 years of Division 1 football. He was symptomatic. He had a number of concussions from which he didn't fully recover. He had difficulty with memory, attention, word finding, confusion, headaches, and difficulty sleeping. He quit football, but it didn't make him better; his symptoms continued to get worse. His cognitive problems eventually forced him to quit college. His symptoms continued to worsen, and he developed depression, impulsivity, and anger. He died at age 25 from an overwhelming infection. When we looked at his 25-year-old brain there was tremendous tau pathology, again right around those blood vessels.[3] We saw it in the frontal lobes, temporal lobes, parietal lobes; this was substantial disease in a 25-year-old. If you can see it with your naked eye, without a microscope, it means there is tremendous disease there. Normally it takes a microscope to make a diagnosis, but in this disease sometimes you don't need one.

Tyler Sash was a 27-year-old who played 2 years for the NFL (Fig. 2.11). He also had symptoms from concussions that didn't resolve. His parents noticed changes in his behavior. He left the NFL after a number of orthopedic issues and surgeries, but he continued to have cognitive problems, including impairment in memory, attention, and executive functioning. He was using narcotics for his chronic pain, and he died from accidental overdose. Here is his brain. He was only 27 years old, and that lesion indicated by the arrow is over an inch long. That is a huge lesion in the frontal lobe of a 27-year-old, a tremendous lesion (Fig. 2.11B). This is what it looked like under the microscope: perivascular tau, the signature lesion of CTE (Fig. 2.11C).

CTE in Football Players From Ages 40 to 82

So what does this disease look like in NFL players? I am going to show you how CTE progresses in NFL players by showing you a series of brains of NFL players who lived past age 40. I am going to show you how this initially focal disease becomes a widespread disease that destroys the primary architecture of the brain. Here is a series of former NFL players by their age at death (Fig. 2.12). There are similarities, but they aren't exactly the same. The patterns of involvement differ slightly, but as one gets older there is greater and greater involvement in different parts of the brain. The medial temporal lobe, including the amygdala and the hippocampus, becomes severely affected, and by the time one is in their late 50s and 60s, there is overwhelming brain disease that can be extraordinarily severe. Even if one just played college football it can be severe at this age. Greg Ploetz died at the age of 66 with stage 4 CTE. He never played in the NFL, just college.

CTE in Other Sports

So it's not just football, it's also soccer.[4] We've seen CTE in older soccer players and we've see CTE in young soccer players who have had the pathognomonic brain lesion. This individual, who died at the age of 29, played only soccer (no other contact sports) (Fig. 2.13). He started playing in grade school and then in high school, college, and a semiprofessional league. He died of amyotrophic lateral sclerosis (ALS), and he is one of the 17 cases in our series of individuals who had both CTE and ALS. We've always thought that this ALS is not real ALS—this is a motor neuron disease caused by CTE. We are having trouble proving it—we have a lot of skeptics—but that's where we are with this concept of CTE and trauma sometimes causing a motor neuron disease.

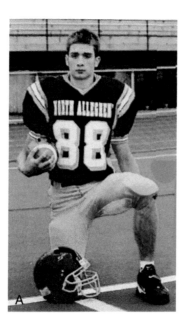

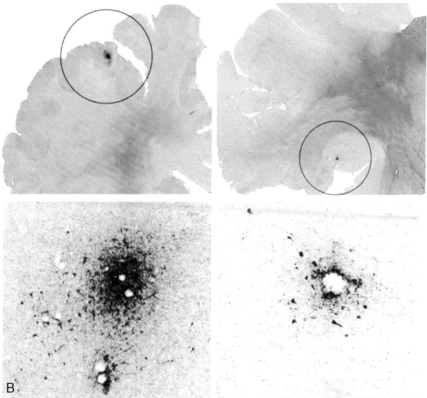

FIG. 2.9 Eric Pelly, an 18-year-old high school football and rugby player. Death occurred 10 days after his fourth concussion. **(A)** Photograph of Eric Pelly. **(B)** Pathology shows stage I CTE. (Figure courtesy of Dr. McKee.)

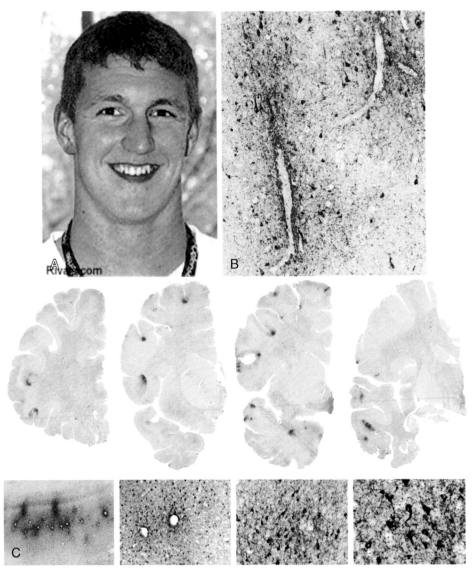

FIG. 2.10 Michael Keck, A 25-year-old college football player, died with symptomatic stage II CTE. **(A)** Photo from college. **(B)** Evidence of stage II CTE. Note that it is easy to see the brown-staining tau in the depths of the sulci. (Images courtesy of Dr. McKee.)

CTE also occurs in hockey players like in Derek Boogaard (Fig. 2.14), but there are many others. We know it happens in military veterans, whether from blast exposure or repetitive head trauma from a variety of other exposures.

CRITICAL QUESTIONS IN CTE

I've shown you much of what we know about the pathology of CTE. So what questions do we need to answer in order to do something about this disease? Here are 10 questions that I think are important:

1. How common is CTE? How many people have it?
2. How can we diagnose CTE during life?
3. Do concussions matter or is it prolonged exposure to repetitive mild trauma/subconcussions?
4. Could anybody get CTE? Or are there genetic susceptibility factors?
5. Are young brains more susceptible to CTE? What about women?

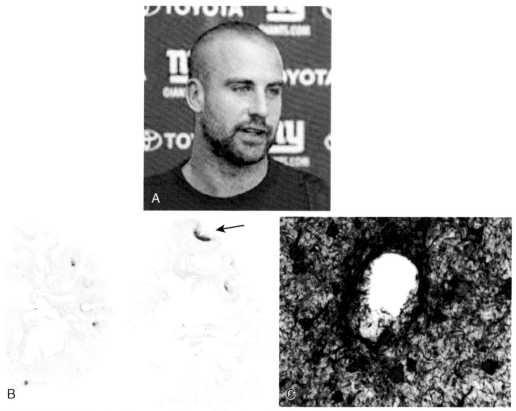

FIG. 2.11 Tyler Sash, a 27-year-old former NFL player. He played football for 16 years, 2 years in the NFL, safety and kick coverage. He had 20 concussions, and he had persistent symptoms from his last concussion. He was noted to be more aggressive and anxious. **(A)** Photo from an NFL press conference. **(B)** Low-power view, with *arrow* showing a brown-staining CTE lesion over 1 inch long. **(C)** Classic perivascular lesion of CTE. (Figure courtesy of Dr. McKee.)

6. How does CTE start in the brain?
7. Once CTE is started, how does it spread in the brain even in the absence of trauma?
8. What is the connection between CTE and motor neuron disease?
9. Does trauma or CTE provoke other neurodegenerations like Alzheimer's and Parkinson's diseases?
10. What are the treatments for CTE?

Answering these questions is important because we need treatments and we need to bring hope to these people and their families who are worried. I am going to quickly go through some of the answers that we are starting to come up with.

How Common Is CTE? How Many People Have It?

Autopsy studies will not tell us how common this disease is. We need to diagnose this disease during life to know how common it is. We need large-scale, long-standing, prospective studies following thousands of student athletes to fully answer this question.

How Can We Diagnose CTE During Life?

We need studies to work toward diagnosing CTE during life. The kind of studies that Dr. Robert Stern is doing (Chapter 3), and that the Department of Veterans Affairs is talking about funding. For example, a prospective study that follows 1000 athletes from not just military academies and colleges but from other high schools and colleges throughout the United States, and follows them for 20 to 35 years to see how they are functioning and if they get CTE. A study like that will help us to understand how and when it starts. We and others are looking at ways to diagnose CTE during life. Other people at this conference will be talking about

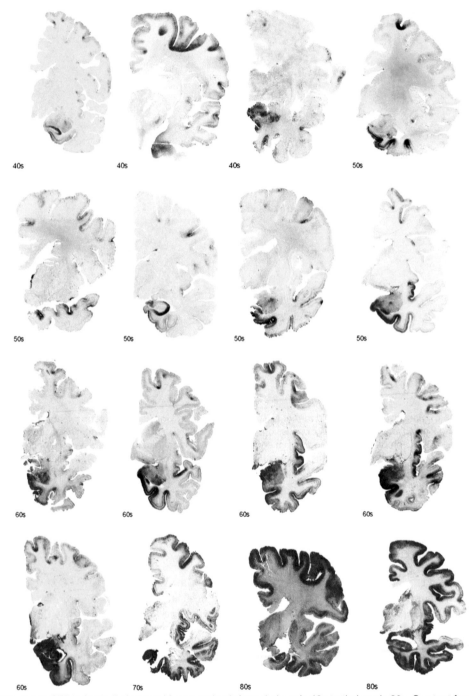

FIG. 2.12 CTE in football players with age at death from their early 40s to their early 80s. See text for details. (Figure courtesy of Dr. McKee.)

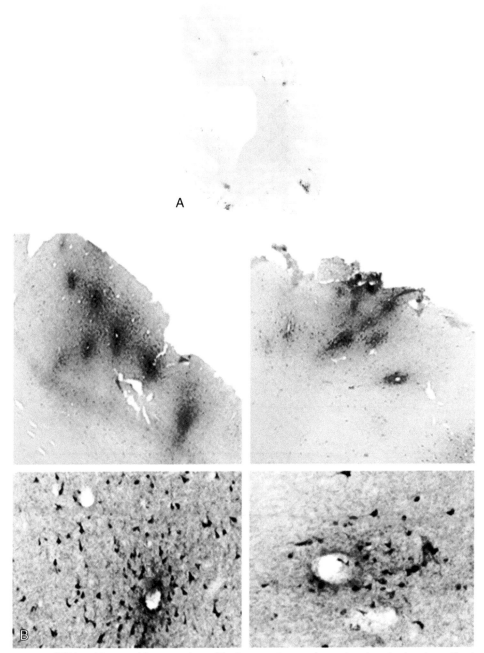

FIG. 2.13 CTE in a 29-year-old soccer player. The images show perivascular phospho-tau deposition in the depths of the sulci. **(A)** Unmagnified. **(B)** Top panels, low power; bottom panels, high power. (Figure courtesy of Dr. McKee.)

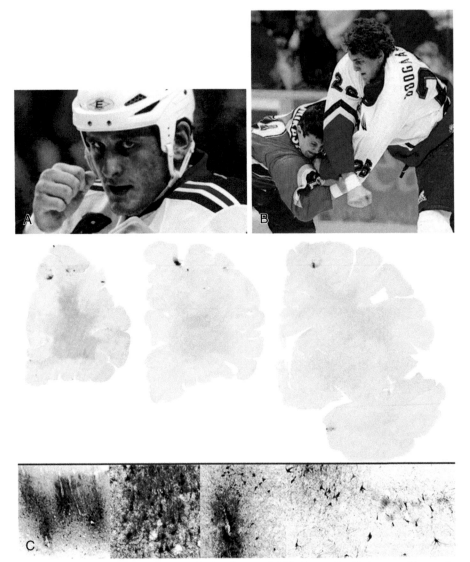

FIG. 2.14 Derek Boogaard was a National Hockey League (NHL) player who died at age 28 years from OxyContin and alcohol and was found to have stage II CTE. **(A** and **B)** Photographs of Boogaard playing hockey. **(C)** Phospho-tau staining showing perivascular lesions at the depths of the sulci in stage II CTE. (Figure courtesy of Dr. McKee.)

these issues, but there are some promising techniques being developed, including imaging[5] (Fig. 2.15) and blood tests.[6]

Do Concussions Matter or Is It Prolonged Exposure to Repetitive Mild Trauma/Subconcussions?

A recent study we conducted with 93 former high school and collegiate football players found that an index measuring their cumulative head impacts was able to predict their self-reported cognitive impairment, depression, apathy, and behavioral dysregulation.[7] From studies like this one we believe it is not concussions, but prolonged exposure to repetitive mild trauma, that matters.

Could Anybody Get CTE? Or Are There Genetic Susceptibility Factors?

We need to find out more about who gets CTE and who doesn't after exposures like playing football. Are there

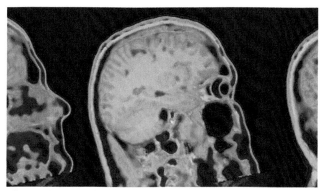

FIG. 2.15 PET imaging studies are using tau ligands in an attempt to diagnose CTE during life. Images show possible CTE pathology (brown/orange color in brain) in a 39-year-old retired NFL player showing progressive emotional lability, irritability, and decline in executive function. (With permission from Dickstein DL, et al. Cerebral [18F]T807/AV1451 retention pattern in clinically probable CTE resembles pathognomonic distribution of CTE tauopathy. *Translational Psychiatry*. September 27, 2016;6(9):e900.)

genetic factors that make it more likely? Is one more likely to develop CTE if one has an APOE4 allele or an MAPT H1 haplotype? We are just beginning to find answers to these questions.

Are Young Brains More Susceptible to CTE? What About Women?

We don't yet know for sure if young brains are more susceptible to CTE, but work that Dr. Julie Stamm and Dr. Stern have conducted found that in NFL players there was more severe late-life cognitive impairment if their first exposure to football was under 12 years of age.[8] These individuals also had more severe diffusion tensor imaging abnormalities in the corpus callosum of their brains.[9] In addition, a new paper just released found that in a single season of youth football with 8- to 13-year-olds, there was a statistically significant relationship between head impact exposure and change in fractional anisotropy of the major white-matter tracts in the brain in the absence of clinically diagnosed concussions.[10] That means these kids' brains may be damaged by just one season of football.

How about women? Does CTE occur in women? We know it has been reported in women. It was diagnosed in an autistic woman who banged her head and died at the age of 24; she had CTE.[11] It was seen in an abused woman who was assaulted for many years; she died with CTE.[12] In our experience, we haven't seen CTE in women. We have had four women brain donors and they were all negative. But we know women are predisposed to concussions, it takes longer for women to recover from concussions, they have more symptoms, and they have a higher rate of

concussions when playing the same sports as men: soccer 2.1 times greater; basketball 1.7 times greater; softball (women) 3.2 times greater than baseball (men). If concussions are related to CTE then these factors may make women more likely to get CTE given the same contact exposures.

How Does CTE Start in the Brain?

We need to know where CTE starts in the brain and how it starts. We need to understand, and answering this question is where pathology and brain donors come in. We are learning from cases like 21-year-old Owen Thomas and 25-year-old Zachary Langston, both of whom committed suicide.

We know it starts in perivascular lesions. So we know how it starts, we just don't know exactly why it starts. There is a lot of attention to the perivascular lesions, including what makes up the normal brain perivascular anatomy, what kind of cells are there, whether there is inflammation, and whether there is breakdown of the blood-brain barrier.

Here are some of the questions we are trying to answer. What kind of tau is there? Is there a special kind of tau in CTE? Does that perivascular lesion affect small blood vessels that are arterioles or is it more on the venous side, the venules? Does the tau accumulate in the nerve cells (neurons) or the astrocytes? What part of the neuron does it accumulate in: the axon, the cell body, or the dendrite? Is there a breakdown of the blood-brain barrier? Are there changes to clearance of substances in the brain, changes to the glymphatic clearance system? Is there a breakdown of the system that would normally get rid of this toxic tau protein? Is the tau pathology associated with neuroinflammation?

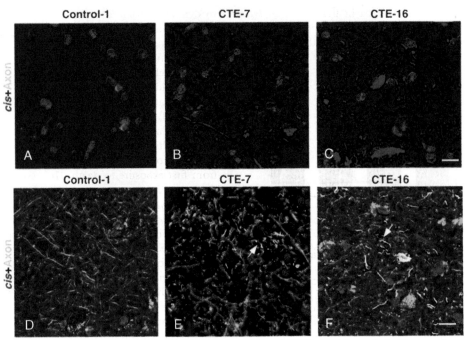

FIG. 2.16 *cis*-Phospho-tau (p-tau) is present in human cases of CTE but not in controls. Top panels: samples stain red for *cis*-p-tau. Bottom panels: samples stain green for *trans*-p-tau. Note the red-staining *cis*-p-tau is present in the CTE cases (**B** and **C**) but not in controls (panel **A**). Green-staining *trans*-p-tau is present in CTE cases (**E** and **F**) and controls (**D**). (With permission from Kondo A, et al. Antibody against early driver of neurodegeneration *cis* P-tau blocks brain injury and tauopathy. *Nature.* July 23, 2015;523(7561):431–436. http://dx.doi.org/10.1038/nature14658. PMID: 26176913.)

Is inflammation driving this pathology? Is inflammation stoking the fire of the pathology? Do these injuries change what is happening in the brain? Is natural aging making the tau pathology much worse? These are just some of the questions that need to be answered.

We are beginning to learn some of the answers to these questions. We know that the tau is distinct. It is not like the tau in Alzheimer's disease. Although it shares many of the same isoforms, it also has different isoforms.[13] We do know a tau isoform called *cis*-phospho-tau may actually drive the pathology (Fig. 2.16). If you use an antibody against this form of tau in experimental animals, it actually suppresses the amount of tau that is deposited as the animal ages.[14]

We know that most of the perivascular lesions are arterioles, because of the staining of the smooth muscle actin along with tau pathology. Once in a while there are venules with tau pathology, but that seems to be more related to astrocytic pathology. We know from Dr. Russ Huber's work that the perivascular lesions are mostly neuronal—we see tau in the nerve cells. We also know that most of the neurites involved are

dendrites. We know that around the perivascular lesion the astrocytes die off or move away. When you look at the perivascular lesion you will see how the astrocytes are actually away from the blood vessel. We're trying to understand what that means.

We know that there is a change to the blood-brain barrier; there is leakiness in the barrier and this finding has been seen at other centers.[15] We've also seen the breakdown of the blood-brain barrier in Dr. Huber's work. He has seen proteins deposited in the brain that shouldn't be there, like fibrinogen, and we know that the fibrinogen actually colocalizes with the tau deposition. We also know that there is a loss of aquaporin-4 and dysfunction of the glymphatic clearance system in CTE from earlier studies.

Here is a new study from Dr. John Cherry and Dr. Stein, very important work that came out 2 days ago.[16] You can see in Fig. 2.17 that inflammation is a key factor here. We see a significant increase in inflammatory cells and inflammation before you even get to CTE pathology. So those repetitive hits to the head start inflammation happening in the brain. Inflammation is trying

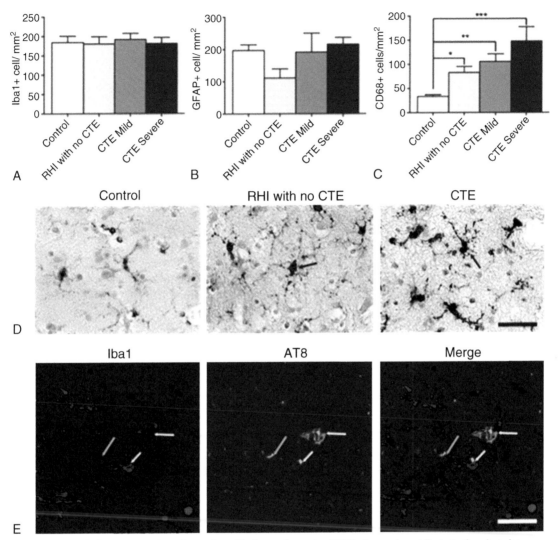

FIG. 2.17 Inflammatory microglia are found in the perivascular CTE lesion and contribute to the phospho-tau (p-tau) pathology. Panel C shows that there is an increase in neuroinflammation in CTE and repetitive head injury (RHI) without CTE. Panel D shows an increase in activated microglia and panel E shows that inflammatory cells (Iba1 positive) and p-tau (AT8 positive) colocalize together. (With permission from Cherry JD, et al. Microglial neuroinflammation contributes to tau accumulation in chronic traumatic encephalopathy. *Acta Neuropathologica Communications*. October 28, 2016;4(1):112. PMID: 27793189.)

to repair the injury, but when it gets out of whack it seems to make the injury worse. In CTE, inflammation goes up substantially as the tau pathology increases. Then tau pathology seems to drive more inflammation, and it becomes a vicious cycle of tau and inflammation making the pathology progressively worse.

So here is what we know so far about how CTE starts in the brain. We know that arterioles are damaged. Neurons are damaged around the arterioles. The p-tau accumulates primarily in the cell body in neurofibrillary tangles and in neurites. Astrocytes around the arteriole mostly disappear, and some accumulate tau. There is loss of blood-brain barrier integrity, causing leakage of proteins. There is tremendous microglia inflammation that promotes further tau accumulation, and we know that there is a loss of aquaporin-4 and breakdown of the glymphatic clearance system of the brain.

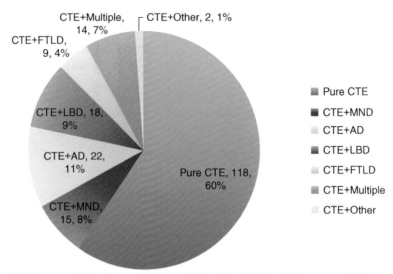

FIG. 2.18 In 198 cases of chronic traumatic encephalopathy (CTE) in athletes, comorbid neurodegeneration was observed in 40%. *AD*, Alzheimer's disease; *FTLD*, frontotemporal lobar degeneration; *LBD*, lewy body disease; *MND*, motor neuron disease. (Figure courtesy of Dr. McKee.)

Once CTE Is Started, How Does It Spread in the Brain Even in the Absence of Trauma?

We need to figure out how CTE spreads in the brain and we are starting to look at possible mechanisms. Prion templating of p-tau is probably the most popular theory, and there is a publication in the works that supports this hypothesis. Glymphatic channel dysfunction with loss of p-tau clearance is definitely a possibility, and more work needs to be done on that topic. We also need to look at blood-brain barrier breakdown and persistent inflammation as possible causes of worsening p-tau accumulation. It would be wonderful if we could control or at least modify CTE by treating with antiinflammatory medications.

Does Trauma or CTE Provoke Other Neurodegenerations Like Alzheimer's and Parkinson's Diseases?

We know that CTE is associated in about 40% of cases with other neurodegenerations (Fig. 2.18), and Dr. Stein will talk about that tomorrow, and how trauma and CTE seem to aggravate other things like Parkinson's and frontal temporal dementia (Chapter 8). CTE starts breaking down a lot of pathways when it affects the brain.

What Are the Treatments for CTE?

We will hear from Dr. Goldstein about mouse models of brain trauma: the blast models and concussion models. Those are what we need to concentrate on if we are going to develop treatments, because we have to come up with something that is helping the animal not get CTE before we can apply it to humans.

SUMMARY

This is how I put all the pieces together to understand CTE (Fig. 2.19). Mild repetitive brain trauma causes an increase in tau. Tau accumulates to the point where the brain can no longer compensate. You start getting behavioral changes, inflammation, and breakdown of the blood-brain barrier. Maybe certain genetic factors make the disease worse, maybe other exposures (like steroids or drugs) make it worse—we don't know. As the disease progresses you get memory loss, other cognitive changes, and then finally dementia.

We do need to do something about this disease. I don't know about you, but I can't stand it when I hear on the news that someone is worried about getting CTE. We are currently so helpless in what we can do for them. I want to bring these athletes who have expressed concern about CTE—Jim McMahon, Tony Dorsett, Brett Farvre, and Ted Johnson—some hope and, more importantly, I want to be able to say we stopped this disease from happening. Young kids coming to the brain bank, dying from suicide and other causes with the earliest stages of CTE, it has to stop.

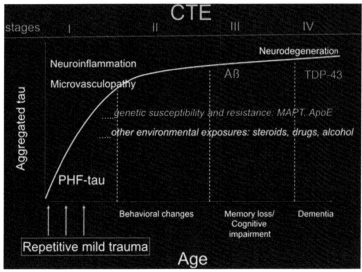

FIG. 2.19 Our current understanding of CTE. See text for details. (Figure courtesy of Dr. McKee.)

I want to thank everyone on my team for all the work that they do. I'm very fortunate that I have a great team. I wouldn't be able to do this work without all of them.

DISCLOSURES

Ann C. McKee has received funding from the NFL, WWE, and the Andlinger Foundation and is a member of the Mackey-White Committee of the NFL Players Association. She receives travel expenses and honoraria for educational lectures.

REFERENCES

1. McKee AC, Cairns NJ, Dickson DW, et al. The first NINDS/NIBIB consensus meeting to define neuropathological criteria for the diagnosis of chronic traumatic encephalopathy. *Acta Neuropathologica.* January 2016;131(1):75–86. http://dx.doi.org/10.1007/s00401-015-1515-z. PMID: 26667418.
2. Bieniek KF, Ross OA, Cormier KA, et al. Chronic traumatic encephalopathy pathology in a neurodegenerative disorders brain bank. *Acta Neuropathologica.* December 2015;130(6):877–889. http://dx.doi.org/10.1007/s00401-015-1502-4. PMID: 26518018.
3. Mez J, Solomon TM, Daneshvar DH, Stein TD, McKee AC. Pathologically confirmed chronic traumatic encephalopathy in a 25-year-old former college football player. *JAMA Neurology.* March 2016;73(3):353–355. http://dx.doi.org/10.1001/jamaneurol.2015.3998. No abstract available. PMID: 26747562.
4. Hales C, Neill S, Gearing M, Cooper D, Glass J, Lah J. Late-stage CTE pathology in a retired soccer player with dementia. *Neurology.* December 9, 2014;83(24):2307–2309.

http://dx.doi.org/10.1212/WNL.0000000000001081. No abstract available. PMID: 25378682.
5. Dickstein DL, Pullman MY, Fernandez C, et al. Cerebral [18F]T807/AV1451 retention pattern in clinically probable CTE resembles pathognomonic distribution of CTE tauopathy. *Translational Psychiatry.* September 27, 2016;6(9):e900. http://dx.doi.org/10.1038/tp.2016.175. PMID: 27676441.
6. Stern RA, Tripodis Y, Baugh CM, et al. Preliminary study of plasma exosomal tau as a potential biomarker for chronic traumatic encephalopathy. *The Journal of Alzheimer's Disease.* 2016;51(4):1099–1109. http://dx.doi.org/10.3233/JAD-151028. PMID: 26890775.
7. Montenigro PH, Alosco ML, Martin BM, et al. Cumulative head impact exposure predicts later-life depression, apathy, executive dysfunction, and cognitive impairment in former high school and college football players. *The Journal of Neurotrauma.* March 30, 2016. [Epub ahead of print]. PMID: 27029716.
8. Stamm JM, Bourlas AP, Baugh CM, et al. Age of first exposure to football and later-life cognitive impairment in former NFL players. *Neurology.* March 17, 2015;84(11):1114–1120. http://dx.doi.org/10.1212/WNL.0000000000001358. PMID: 25632088.
9. Stamm JM, Koerte IK, Muehlmann M, et al. Age at first exposure to football is associated with altered corpus callosum white matter microstructure in former professional football players. *Journal of Neurotrauma.* November 15, 2015;32(22):1768–1776. http://dx.doi.org/10.1089/neu.2014.3822. PMID: 26200068.
10. Bahrami N, Sharma D, Rosenthal S, et al. Subconcussive head impact exposure and white matter tract changes over a single season of youth Football. *Radiology.* December 2016;281(3):919–926. PMID: 27775478.

11. Hof PR, Knabe R, Bovier P, Bouras C. Neuropathological observations in a case of autism presenting with self-injury behavior. *Acta Neuropathologica.* 1991;82(4):321–326. PMID: 1759563.

12. Roberts GW, Whitwell HL, Acland PR, Bruton CJ. Dementia in a punch-drunk wife. *Lancet.* April 14, 1990;335(8694):918–919. No abstract available. PMID: 1970008.

13. Kanaan NM, Cox K, Alvarez VE, Stein TD, Poncil S, McKee AC. Characterization of early pathological tau conformations and phosphorylation in chronic traumatic encephalopathy. *Journal of Neuropathology and Experimental Neurology.* January 2016;75(1):19–34. PMID: 26671985.

14. Kondo A, Shahpasand K, Mannix R, et al. Antibody against early driver of neurodegeneration cis P-tau blocks brain injury and tauopathy. *Nature.* July 23, 2015;523(7561):431–436. http://dx.doi.org/10.1038/nature14658. PMID: 26176913.

15. Doherty CP, O'Keefe E, Wallace E, et al. Blood-brain barrier dysfunction as a hallmark pathology in chronic traumatic encephalopathy. *The Journal of Neuropathology & Experimental Neurology.* July 2016;75(7):656–662. http://dx.doi.org/10.1093/jnen/nlw036. PMID: 27245243.

16. Cherry JD, Tripodis Y, Alvarez VE, et al. Microglial neuroinflammation contributes to tau accumulation in chronic traumatic encephalopathy. *Acta Neuropathologica Communications.* October 28, 2016;4(1):112. PMID: 27793189.

FURTHER READING

McKee AC, Stern RA, Nowinski CJ, et al. The spectrum of disease in chronic traumatic encephalopathy. *Brain.* January 2013;136(Pt 1):43–64. http://dx.doi.org/10.1093/brain/aws307. Erratum in: Brain. 2013 Oct;136(Pt 10):e255.

CHAPTER 3

Chronic Traumatic Encephalopathy: Clinical Presentation and Diagnostic Criteria

ROBERT A. STERN • MICHAEL L. ALOSCO

INTRODUCTION

It is an honor to be here, and it is a tremendous honor to be surrounded by the family members of our legacy donors. Yesterday, I had the unbelievable experience of being able to spend time with these family members. These are the families that we have performed telephone interviews with in order to study chronic traumatic encephalopathy (CTE) and examine how this disease affects individuals and their families. To be surrounded by individuals who have been affected by CTE has been one of the most powerful experiences in my life. I would like to emphasize the strength and generosity of these family members and all who donated their brains for research to our Center. The contributions of the families, combined with Dr. Ann McKee's groundbreaking work describing the neuropathology of CTE, have led to an unbelievable impact on public awareness, public policy, and scientific research.

CTE: WHAT WE NEED TO KNOW

The public tends to believe we know more about CTE than we actually do. For several years, I have been saying that we are in the infancy of our knowledge of CTE. But, I now think we are in the toddlerhood of this scientific journey. As described by Dr. McKee in Chapter 2, one of the key questions in the emerging field of CTE is in regards to prevalence; is CTE common? We don't know how common CTE is, but it has the potential to be a major public health issue. We also need to determine why some individuals develop CTE and others do not. All neuropathologically confirmed cases of CTE to date have had a history of repetitive head impacts (RHI), suggesting that exposure to RHI is necessary for the development of CTE. However, RHI is not sufficient, given that many individuals with a history of RHI do *not* develop CTE. What are the risk factors that interact with

exposure to RHI to trigger the pathogenesis of CTE? Is there a genetic predisposition that may affect the risk for developing CTE? Dr. Jesse Mez, in Chapter 7, will describe what we currently know about the genetics of CTE. In addition to genetics, perhaps there are individual differences in head trauma exposure that may affect the risk for developing CTE, including severity of head trauma, type of head trauma, duration of RHI exposure, total number of hits, interval rest between hits, to name a few. Head trauma exposure risk factors of particular interest to my colleagues and me at Boston University (BU) include age of first exposure to RHI as well as the cumulative number of hits.

HISTORY AND ANTHROPOLOGY OF REPETITIVE HEAD IMPACTS

I would like to discuss briefly the history and anthropology of RHI. Humans have been in existence for approximately 200,000 years, and there has never been a time period when humans have been exposed to repetitive concussive and subconcussive blows to the head, until boxing became a common sport in the 19th and 20th centuries. We've known about the negative neurological effects of boxing since the early 1900s, when terms such as "punch drunk" and "dementia pugilistica" (later termed CTE) were first used.[1,2] However, it is likely that the repetitive blows to the head in boxing began to increase dramatically with the advent of the padded boxing glove in the middle 20th century. The padded glove was meant to reduce injuries to the hands of the boxer throwing the punch. However, it is likely that an additional outcome was the increase in the number of repetitive blows to the head, due to the diminished pain incurred by both the individual throwing the punch and the recipient of the blow. American tackle football began in the late 19th century. It was originally played without any protective headgear and then small leather helmets were used. However, it wasn't until the 1950s and 1960s that hard plastic helmets with face masks were used. The helmets were developed to prevent skull fractures (which they did and continue to do), but they also allowed individuals to hit their head repeatedly against their opponent without feeling pain, creating a sense of invincibility and also portraying minimal safety concerns. In the 1960s and early 1970s, children started to play American tackle football, and Pop Warner youth football became popular nationally. From a public health perspective, the first individuals who played youth football are currently in their late 50s and 60s, and the first individuals who played college football with hard plastic helmets and face masks are currently in their mid-70s. Therefore, in that long history of humankind, it is only in the past 55 to 65 years that our species has been exposed to RHI. Although the epidemiology of CTE is unknown, it is possible that millions of living older adults are currently at high risk for CTE due to their history of exposure to RHI.

LONG-TERM CONSEQUENCES OF REPETITIVE HEAD IMPACT EXPOSURE

The long-term consequences of RHI have been the focus of our research at BU. Of particular concern are the children between the ages of 9 and 12 in the United States that participate in youth tackle football. These children are exposed to RHI during critical periods of neurodevelopment. The time period between 9 and 12 years old is when the brain undergoes tremendous maturation.[3-14] Dr. Julie Stamm, a PhD student of mine and Dr. Martha Shenton's, examined whether RHI during this time window of peak neurodevelopment may increase vulnerability to long-term consequences. Dr. Stamm investigated the association between age of first exposure to tackle football and later-life clinical and neurological outcomes in a sample of former National Football League (NFL) players. Briefly, her results showed that former NFL players who began playing tackle football before age 12 had significantly worse cognitive functioning,[15] as well as microstructural integrity of the anterior corpus callosum,[16] compared to former NFL players who began playing tackle football at 12 or older (see also Chapter 11).

Stamm and colleagues examined only former *professional* football players and did not investigate cumulative hits to the head. Dr. Philip Montenigro, an MD/PhD student of mine, addressed these limitations and used former amateur American football players to develop the cumulative head impact index (CHII). The CHII is

a metric that estimates the total number of hits above a certain *g* force that an individual received throughout their lifetime.[17] Montenigro and colleagues used the CHII to examine the relationship between cumulative lifetime RHI exposure and later-life clinical function in former amateur American football players.[17] The findings showed a dose-response relationship between the total number of hits an amateur football player received and later-life risk for clinical depression measured by the Center for Epidemiologic Studies Depression Scale[18] (Fig. 3.1A), cognitive impairment measured by the Brief Test of Adult Cognition by Telephone[19] (Fig. 3.1B), and behavioral dysregulation measured by the Behavior Rating Inventory of Executive Function, Adult version (BRIEF-A)[20] (Fig. 3.1C). The development of the CHII will facilitate research on RHI and later-life neurological outcomes, including CTE, once it is able to be diagnosed during life.

DIAGNOSIS OF CTE DURING LIFE: THE CRITICAL NEXT STEP

A critical next step is to be able to diagnose CTE during life and differentiate CTE from other causes of cognitive and behavioral changes, including Alzheimer's disease (AD), frontotemporal lobar degeneration (FTLD), posttraumatic stress disorder, depression, and chronic problems associated with traumatic brain injury. Once we can diagnose CTE during life and differentiate it from similar neurological and psychiatric conditions, the incidence and prevalence of CTE can be determined and risk factors can be investigated, including the genetic and head trauma exposure variables previously discussed. In particular, being able to diagnose CTE during life will allow for clinical trials for treatment and prevention to begin. The first step in being able to diagnose CTE during life is to characterize the clinical features. Next, I will discuss what we think the clinical presentation of CTE is at this time, through presentation of two clinical vignettes of autopsy-confirmed cases of CTE. I will then give a brief review of the existing retrospective postmortem data.

Clinical Features of CTE: Case Examples
Case 1
This is the case of Dave Duerson. Mr. Duerson died at the age of 50. He was a well-known player for the Chicago Bears and was on the last Super Bowl–winning Chicago Bears team in 1986. He was a very successful businessperson after he retired from the NFL, but he spiraled downward the last 5 years of his life. He had worsening memory difficulties, was behaviorally out of control, had

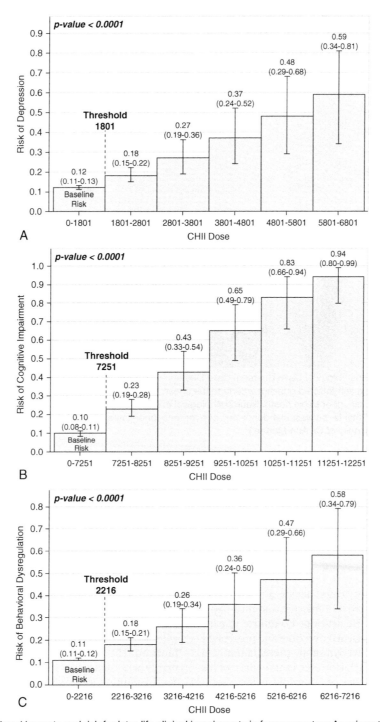

FIG. 3.1 Repetitive head impacts and risk for later-life clinical impairments in former amateur American tackle football players. The x-axis is the total number of lifetime cumulative head impacts. The y-axis is risk for clinical impairment for the following: **(A)** depression as measured by the Center for Epidemiologic Studies Depression Scale, **(B)** objective cognitive function as measured by the Brief Test of Adult Cognition by Telephone, and **(C)** reported behavioral regulation as measured by the Behavioral Regulation Index from the Behavior Rating Inventory of Executive Function, Adult version. For each clinical domain, there is a dose-response relationship with the cumulative head impact index (CHII). (From Montenigro PH, Alosco ML, Martin BM, et al. Cumulative head impact exposure predicts later-life depression, apathy, executive dysfunction, and cognitive impairment in former high school and college football players. *Journal of Neurotrauma*. 2016. http://dx.doi.org/10.1089/neu.2016.4413.)

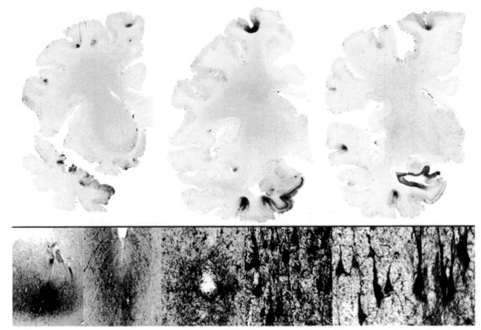

FIG. 3.2 Neuropathology of Dave Duerson. Dave Duerson was a former NFL player who died at the age of 50 years from a self-inflicted gunshot wound to the chest. He had cognitive, behavioral, and mood problems for many years prior to his death. Neuropathological examination of his brain was positive for CTE neuropathology, that is, perivascular deposition of hyperphosphorylated tau at the depths of the cortical sulci. (Figure courtesy of Dr. Ann McKee.)

a short fuse, and was physically abusive with his wife. He lost his business, as well as his marriage. He died by suicide from a self-inflicted gunshot wound to the chest; he chose the chest in order to avoid hurting his brain so that it could be studied. Neuropathological examination of his brain was positive for CTE (Fig. 3.2).

Case 2

This is the case of Barry "Tizza" Taylor, a rugby player from Australia. He played 235 matches and thus had a high exposure to RHI. He developed cognitive impairment in his 50s that worsened over time and progressed to severe dementia. His symptom presentation was remarkably similar to AD. However, examination of his brain showed no evidence of β-amyloid neuropathology, which is a necessary finding in AD. Instead, there was hyperphosphorylated tau throughout his brain, in a pattern consistent with CTE.[21]

Clinical Presentation of CTE: Retrospective Postmortem Data

Based on the previous literature of boxers with dementia pugilistica, and research from our Center,[22] there seemed to be four domains of clinical impairment associated with CTE: (1) *cognitive impairment*, particularly in episodic memory and executive function that progresses to dementia; (2) *mood disturbances*, primarily characterized by depression and hopelessness; (3) *behavioral disturbances*, including impulsivity, explosivity, and aggression; and (4) *parkinsonism*, present in a subset of cases, predominantly the boxers. The literature further suggested two different subtypes in the clinical presentation of CTE. The first presentation involves onset at a young age of mood and behavior problems, with minimal disturbances in cognitive and motor function. The second are individuals who present primarily with deficits in cognitive function at an older age, in addition to motor disturbances occasionally.

To clarify the clinical presentation of CTE, my colleagues and I conducted a study that examined the clinical course and features of 36 deceased contact sport athletes with neuropathologically confirmed CTE, without any other disease present.[23] We conducted extensive semistructured interviews with family members of the deceased and also reviewed available medical records. The clinicians who conducted the clinical

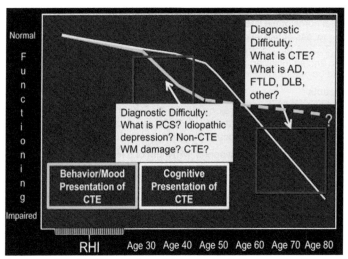

FIG. 3.3 Clinical presentation of CTE and differential diagnosis challenges. *AD*, Alzheimer's disease; *DLB*, dementia due to Lewy body; *FTLD*, frontotemporal lobar degeneration; *PCS*, postconcussion syndrome; *RHI*, repetitive head impacts; *WM*, white matter. (Figure courtesy of Dr. Robert Stern.)

activities were blind to the neuropathology, and the neuropathologists who examined the brains were blind to the clinical histories. Of the 36 contact sport athletes with CTE, 33 were symptomatic. The three who were asymptomatic included a teenager with stage 1 CTE and two others with mild CTE pathology plus a high level of cognitive reserve (e.g., high educational attainment)—potentially representing a key protective factor. Overall, the findings were consistent with the two different initial clinical presentations described above. One of the presentations was that of behavioral and mood changes that began early in life, and the other was of cognitive impairment later in life. We also found that the behavioral and mood group tended to develop cognitive problems later on and that dementia was common in the cognitive group.

Although this study led to an improved understanding of the clinical presentation of CTE, there remain many complexities in terms of differential diagnosis (Fig. 3.3). Decline in behavior and mood function often begins during active exposure to RHI, followed by a sharp decline in the 30s and 40s, years after RHI exposure has ended. The initial changes in behavior and mood could potentially be related to postconcussion syndrome, or from a psychiatric illness (e.g., depression), or from white matter alterations directly due to the brain trauma at the time of exposure. However, the persistence and progression of behavior and mood symptoms over time argues for the presence of a neurodegenerative process, like CTE. In terms of the cognitive

clinical presentation, cognitive symptoms may begin in the 40s, with overt and rapid decline evident in the 50s and 60s. The cognitive decline in the 50s and 60s can often mimic AD and other neurodegenerative diseases such as FTLD or Lewy body dementia. Dr. Andrew Budson describes the similarities and differences between the clinical features of CTE and other neurodegenerative diseases in Chapter 9.

TRAUMATIC ENCEPHALOPATHY SYNDROME

To facilitate differential diagnosis of CTE from similarly presenting neurological and psychiatric conditions, provisional clinical research diagnostic criteria were developed, referred to as traumatic encephalopathy syndrome (TES).[22] It was not referred to as CTE because CTE is a neuropathological entity. TES is a clinical syndrome associated with exposure to RHI that can be a manifestation of various etiologies. TES includes five general criteria, three core clinical features, and nine supportive features (Table 3.1). There are four potential diagnostic variants: TES behavioral/mood variant, TES cognitive variant, TES mixed variant, and TES dementia variant; the dementia variant is further defined by the subtypes present (i.e., cognitive, behavioral/mood, or mixed). The TES criteria were developed based on the state of the literature at that time. Thus, these are provisional criteria that will continue to change as new evidence and findings emerge. If an individual meets the

TABLE 3.1
Traumatic Encephalopathy Syndrome Diagnostic Criteria

A. PUBLISHED GENERAL CRITERIA FOR TRAUMATIC ENCEPHALOPATHY SYNDROME (TES)

All five criteria (1 to 5) must be met for diagnosis

1. History of Multiple Impacts

Types of injuries	Concussion or mTBI. If no other RTBI then minimum of 4 Moderate/severe TBI. If no other RTBI then minimum of 2 Subconcussive trauma
Source of exposures	Contact sports. Minimum of 6 years Military service Other RTBI exposures, e.g., domestic abuse

2. Other Neurological Disorder That Likely Accounts for All Clinical Features

Exclude if	A single TBI Or persistent PCS
Can be present	Substance abuse Posttraumatic stress disorder Mood/anxiety disorders Other neurodegenerative diseases

3. Clinical Features Must Be Present for a Minimum of 12 Months

4. "Core Clinical Features" of TES

At least one must be present	*Cognitive*. Difficulties identified by standardized mental status or cognitive neuropsychological test at least 1.5. STD below normal *Behavioral*. Described as explosive, short fuse, out of control, physically and/or verbally violent. Or intermittent explosive disorder *Mood*. Feeling overly sad, depressed, or hopeless. Or diagnosis of major depressive disorder or persistent depressive disorder

5. "Supportive Features" of TES

At least two must be present	Documented decline (1 year), delayed onset, impulsivity, anxiety, apathy, paranoia, suicidality, headache, motor

B. CRITERIA FOR DIAGNOSTIC SUBTYPES WITH MODIFIERS

1. TES Diagnostic Variants

Select one	"Cognitive"	Cognitive core features without behavioral/mood
	"Behavioral/mood"	Behavioral/mood core features without cognitive
	"Mixed"	Both cognitive and behavioral/mood core features
	"Dementia"	Progressive cognitive core and functional impairment

2. "With Motor Features" Modifier

"With motor features"	Dysarthria, dysgraphia, bradykinesia, tremor, rigidity, gait change, falls, and/or other features of parkinsonism

3. Clinical Course Modifier

Select one	"Stable"	History or tests indicate little if any change
	"Progressive"	Clear indication of progression over 2 years
	"Unknown/inconsistent"	Unknown or inconsistent information

TABLE 3.1
Traumatic Encephalopathy Syndrome Diagnostic Criteria—cont'd

C. CHRONIC TRAUMATIC ENCEPHALOPATHY (CTE) LIKELIHOOD CRITERIA

"Probable CTE"	Does not satisfy criteria for another disorder more consistently	
	Meets classification for any TES variant	
	Progressive course	
	At least one positive "potential bio-marker"	Positive PET tau imaging
		Negative PET amyloid imaging
		Normal β amyloid CSF levels
		Elevated CSF p-tau/tau ratio
		Cavum septum pellucidum
		Cortical thinning or atrophy
"Possible CTE"	May satisfy diagnostic criteria for another disorder	
	Meets classification for any TES variant	
	Progressive course	
	No testing or one negative biomarker except for PET tau	
"Unlikely CTE"	Does not meet general criteria (1 to 5) for TES	
	Or has had negative PET tau imaging	

CSF, cerebrospinal fluid; *mTBI*, mild traumatic brain injury; *PCS*, postconcussion syndrome; *RTBI*, repetitive traumatic brain injury; *STD*, standard deviation; *TBI*, traumatic brain injury.
These are provisional clinical research diagnostic criteria to facilitate clinical research on CTE. They are not intended for clinical use.
Modified from Montenigro PH, Baugh CM, Daneshvar DH, et al. Clinical subtypes of chronic traumatic encephalopathy: literature review and proposed research diagnostic criteria for traumatic encephalopathy syndrome. *Alzheimer's Research and Therapy*. 2014;6(5):68. http://dx.doi.org/10.1186/s13195-014-0068-z.

clinical diagnosis of TES, the next step is to determine whether the etiology is CTE. As part of TES, there are provisional criteria for the likelihood of CTE, with three different categories: "Probable CTE," "Possible CTE," and "Unlikely CTE." To be diagnosed with Probable CTE, the individual must meet the TES criteria, have a progressive clinical course, and have a positive clinical biomarker, consistent with the presence of underlying CTE. These objective biomarkers are currently being developed and are discussed later in this chapter, as well as by Dr. Shenton in Chapter 11, Dr. Blennow in Chapter 10, and Dr. Budson in Chapter 9. The diagnosis of Possible CTE would be assigned if the individual meets the TES criteria but there is no biomarker evidence of CTE. Unlikely CTE is assigned if the individual does not meet the TES criteria or if biomarker findings argue against the likelihood of CTE (e.g., negative tau PET imaging). The following are case examples to illustrate the TES clinical research diagnostic criteria.

Case Example A

This is a 45-year-old man who played American football from age 9 to 22 years old, including 4 years as an offensive lineman at a Division I university. He also played soccer and lacrosse as a youth but discontinued participation in these sports to focus on football. Although he stated that he was never diagnosed with a clinical concussion playing football, after he was provided with a modern definition of concussion, he estimated that he likely experienced 25 to 36 concussions. Following his football career, he worked as an accountant for a small firm. He began to have issues with work performance the last 2 years, as his evaluation reports indicated that he was making careless errors, was less productive, and was argumentative with his boss. His wife stated that he began to have cognitive, mood, and behavioral problems at age 36. His premorbid personality was described to be kind and loving, and this changed to be argumentative and explosive. His behavioral disturbances indeed significantly progressed over the past 5 to 7 years, and he was short fused (including losing his temper with his children). His alcohol consumption also increased the last 2 to 3 years.

He underwent a neuropsychological evaluation that was remarkable for moderate impairments in sustained attention and executive function, with mildly impaired delayed recall of unstructured verbal information. All other cognitive domains were intact. He self-reported mild to moderate symptoms of depression. Instrumental and basic activities of daily living were intact. A brain MRI was read to be remarkable for mild, scattered white matter hyperintensities. Medical history, laboratory findings, and neurological exam were all noncontributory.

He meets criteria for TES mixed variant due to his presentation of cognitive difficulties, behavior and mood changes, and progressive course. Only Possible CTE can be assigned due to lack of biomarker evidence for CTE (scattered white matter hyperintensities are nonspecific).

Case Example B

This case is a 71-year-old former NFL player who underwent numerous evaluations over the past 12 years due to a progressive decline in clinical function. He received multiple diagnoses across these evaluations, including FTLD, AD, and dementia "due to concussions." He began playing football in junior high school and then played at a Division I college. He played in the NFL for 10 years. His primary position in the NFL was linebacker. He worked as an insurance salesperson following retirement from NFL. He had a very successful work career but had to retire at age 61 because of cognitive difficulties, namely, poor decision making and impaired judgment. Per wife, he has been having progressively worsening difficulties with memory and judgment since the age of 59. Multitasking and working with numerical numbers also became problematic for him. In fact, his wife had to assume responsibility of the finances when he was 61 due to his cognitive difficulties. He also could no longer meaningfully engage in his hobbies at age 61. In addition to cognitive problems, he became withdrawn and verbally aggressive at 62. There were instances of physical aggression toward his wife, and she often feared for her safety. There is no history of social disinhibition, symptoms of psychosis, or motor disturbances. His clinical function rapidly declined the last 2 years of his life, and he was fully dependent for all activities of daily living.

Medical history is remarkable for myocardial infarction (age 54), hypertension, hyperlipidemia, and shoulder surgeries. There was no family history of dementia. Neurological evaluations revealed disorientation (to time and place), perseveration, and inability to recall recent or current events. Motor examination was within normal limits. His Mini Mental State Examination score was 10. His Clinical Dementia Rating scale score was 2.0. Neuropsychological evaluation revealed severe impairments in episodic memory and executive functions. Other cognitive domains were largely intact. Brain MRI was read to be positive for severe global atrophy (including enlarged ventricles), with marked hippocampal and amygdala atrophy, and a cavum septum pellucidum (CSP). The CSP was a notable finding because a majority of neuropathologically confirmed cases of CTE have an opening of a sheath between the ventricles, known as a CSP (see Chapters 1, 9, and 11). An amyloid PET scan, an FDA-approved scan for AD

to determine whether there are amyloid plaques in the brain, showed minimal uptake. This individual meets criteria for TES dementia, mixed type. The etiology of Probable CTE can be assigned because of biomarker evidence for CTE neuropathology, including a CSP, severe brain atrophy including of the hippocampi, and a negative amyloid PET scan.

These case examples illustrate the provisional TES criteria, with emphasis on the word *provisional*. It is still not possible to diagnose CTE during life, as the clinical utility of the TES criteria remains unknown and validated available objective biomarkers of CTE do not yet exist.

NEED FOR OBJECTIVE IN VIVO BIOMARKERS

There is a need for the development and validation of objective biomarkers that can support a Probable CTE diagnosis. Biomarkers can provide accurate preclinical detection, which is important because, like AD, the pathophysiology of CTE likely begins years and even decades before symptoms begin. If CTE is a progressive condition, it is critical to develop disease-modifying treatments (e.g., anti-tau agents) and to initiate them early in the disease course prior to the destruction of brain tissue. CTE may begin with initial preclinical focal phosphorylated tau around the blood vessels and at the depths of the sulci. With time, the individual progresses through the clinical stage of TES without dementia. With continued progression, functional problems begin and dementia ensues. Initiation of treatment as early as possible is essential, in order to prevent the symptoms from ever developing or to slow the symptom course of the disease. In order for treatments to be developed and initiated early, we need to be able to detect CTE early during life through the use of biomarkers.

Diagnosing and Evaluating Traumatic Encephalopathy Using Clinical Tests

As in AD, the combination of biomarkers and clinical evaluation will lead to an accurate in vivo diagnosis of CTE. Diagnosing and Evaluating Traumatic Encephalopathy Using Clinical Tests (DETECT) was the first grant funded by the National Institutes of Health (NIH) for the study of CTE, despite knowing about CTE since the 1920s. The goal of DETECT was to develop biomarkers for CTE and identify its clinical features. One hundred symptomatic former NFL players at high risk for CTE and approximately 30 same-age asymptomatic males without head trauma or a history of participation in contact sports were recruited for DETECT. Former NFL players were between 40 and 69 years old and played positions with the greatest exposure to RHI. In addition, all former NFL players recruited must have endorsed symptoms of mood, behavior, and/or cognitive functioning at the time of the study enrollment. As part of the DETECT protocol, subjects completed state-of-the-art neuroimaging techniques, in addition to lumbar puncture, blood draw for DNA and genetic analysis, neurological evaluation, neuropsychological testing, neuropsychiatric examination, and clinical history interviews. When DETECT began, there were no measures of blood or brain tau on the horizon; we need to have a tool that can detect the tau that Dr. McKee has been describing.[21] Data collection for DETECT finished approximately 1 year ago, and has resulted in several preliminary published studies,[15,16,24-27] with several more studies being completed.

Preliminary biomarker findings

Dr. Shenton from Brigham and Woman's Hospital, a collaborator on the DETECT project, discusses the neuroimaging findings from DETECT in Chapter 11. Findings from DETECT demonstrate that a cavum septum pellucidum, found in the majority of cases of neuropathologically diagnosed CTE, is very common in former NFL players and may serve as a potential biomarker for CTE.[26] A study (under review at the time of this writing) highlights the potential utility of magnetic resonance spectroscopy as a possible method to detect CTE in life through examination of neurochemistry. As discussed by Dr. Shenton in Chapter 11, CTE may be associated with unique patterns of volume loss on MRI. The use of PET scans that can detect abnormal tau in vivo will be essential and will likely serve as the gold standard for detecting CTE. Fluid biomarkers that can assess for the presence of CTE neuropathology may also have key and more practical (relative to PET imaging) clinical utility.[25,27] Fluid biomarkers are discussed by Dr. Blennow in Chapter 10. All kinds of new and exciting biomarker research in CTE is happening and will continue to progress with the recently funded NIH/National Institute of Neurological Disorders and Stroke (NINDS) study (U01NS093334), entitled Diagnostics, Imaging, And Genetics Network for the Objective Study & Evaluation of Chronic Traumatic Encephalopathy (DIAGNOSE CTE) Research Project.

DIAGNOSE CTE RESEARCH PROJECT

The DIAGNOSE CTE Research Project is a $16 million NINDS-funded, 7-year, multisite study, with four Principal Investigators: Robert A. Stern, PhD (contact PI); Jeffrey Cummings, MD; Eric Reiman, MD; and Martha Shenton, MD. DIAGNOSE CTE involves collaborating institutions across the country, and subjects are already being examined at the four different evaluation sites, which include Arizona (Mayo Clinic-Scottsdale), Boston (BU School of Medicine), Las Vegas (Cleveland Clinic Lou Ruvo Center for Brain Health), and New York (New York University Langone Medical Center). This research project involves 50 collaborators and 10 research institutions. There is an advisory board of remarkable individuals, including scientific thought leaders and a member of the Pro Football Hall of Fame. The conduct of the DIAGNOSE CTE project is overseen by specific "Teams" of investigators (Fig. 3.4) to address all of the unique complexities involved in the comprehensive clinical study of CTE.

Diagnose CTE Research Project: Methods and Specific Aims

The specific aims of DIAGNOSE CTE include:
1. To collect and analyze neuroimaging and fluid biomarkers for the in vivo detection of CTE.
2. To characterize the clinical presentation of CTE.
3. To examine the progression of CTE over a 3-year period.
4. To refine and validate diagnostic criteria for the clinical diagnosis of CTE.
5. To investigate genetic and head impact exposure risk factors for CTE.
6. To share project data with researchers across the country and abroad.

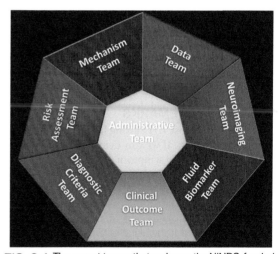

FIG. 3.4 The expert teams that make up the NINDS-funded Diagnostics, Imaging, And Genetics Network for the Objective Study & Evaluation of Chronic Traumatic Encephalopathy (DIAGNOSE CTE) research project. DIAGNOSE CTE involves 50 collaborators and 10 research institutions across the country. Expert teams were developed to address all of the unique complexities involved in the comprehensive study of CTE.

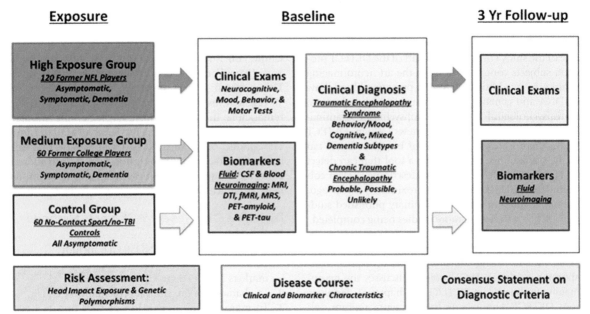

FIG. 3.5 DIAGNOSE CTE research project study design overview.

The design of the project (Fig. 3.5) involves a comprehensive baseline examination of 240 men, ages 45 to 74, including former NFL players, former college football players, and controls without history of contact sports or brain trauma. Subjects are seen again for a 3-year follow-up. The examinations include state-of-the art structural, functional, and molecular neuroimaging, as well as lumbar puncture and blood draws for extensive fluid biomarker measurement, neuropsychological and neuropsychiatric evaluations, neurological examination, and genetics studies.

CONCLUDING REMARKS

Once we can diagnose CTE during life, clinical trials for treatment can begin. If we can detect CTE early in the disease course, prior to symptom onset, we can conduct clinical trials for prevention. We are at an exciting and important time in the study of CTE. In these next few years we will likely see an increased understanding of the underlying neuropathogenetic mechanism of CTE, as well as increased knowledge of the RHI and genetic factors involved in the development of CTE. We will have accurate methods of detecting and diagnosing the disease during life. And, we will begin to have interventions to treat, slow down, and even prevent the symptoms of this disease.

Thank you to all of the individuals who have volunteered as research participants and to my colleagues

and staff who conduct the research and devote their time and energy to helping improve our understanding on CTE. Thank you to the institutes and centers that have been providing funding for our clinical research. Thank you all very much.

REFERENCES

1. Martland HS. Punch drunk. *JAMA*. 1928;91(15):1103–1107.
2. Millspaugh JA. Dementia pugilistica. *United States Naval Medical Bulletin*. 1937;35:297–303.
3. Caviness Jr VS, Kennedy DN, Richelme C, Rademacher J, Filipek PA. The human brain age 7-11 years: a volumetric analysis based on magnetic resonance images. *Cerebral Cortex*. 1996;6(5):726–736.
4. Chugani HT, Phelps ME, Mazziotta JC. Positron emission tomography study of human brain functional development. *Annals of Neurology*. 1987;22(4):487–497. http://dx.doi.org/10.1002/ana.410220408.
5. Courchesne E, Chisum HJ, Townsend J, et al. Normal brain development and aging: quantitative analysis at in vivo MR imaging in healthy volunteers. *Radiology*. 2000;216(3): 672–682. http://dx.doi.org/10.1148/radiology.216.3.r00au 37672.
6. Epstein HT. Stages of increased cerebral blood flow accompany stages of rapid brain growth. *Brain and Development*. 1999;21(8):535–539.
7. Giedd JN. The teen brain: insights from neuroimaging. *The Journal of Adolescent Health*. 2008;42(4):335–343. http://dx.doi.org/10.1016/j.jadohealth.2008.01.007.

8. Giedd JN, Blumenthal J, Jeffries NO, et al. Brain development during childhood and adolescence: a longitudinal MRI study. *Nature Neuroscience.* 1999;2(10):861–863. http://dx.doi.org/10.1038/13158.

9. Lebel C, Walker L, Leemans A, Phillips L, Beaulieu C. Microstructural maturation of the human brain from childhood to adulthood. *Neuroimage.* 2008;40(3):1044–1055. http://dx.doi.org/10.1016/j.neuroimage.2007.12.053.

10. Shaw P, Greenstein D, Lerch J, et al. Intellectual ability and cortical development in children and adolescents. *Nature.* 2006;440(7084):676–679. http://dx.doi.org/10.1038/nature04513.

11. Shaw P, Kabani NJ, Lerch JP, et al. Neurodevelopmental trajectories of the human cerebral cortex. *The Journal of Neuroscience.* 2008;28(14):3586–3594. http://dx.doi.org/10.1523/JNEUROSCI.5309-07.2008.

12. Snook L, Paulson LA, Roy D, Phillips L, Beaulieu C. Diffusion tensor imaging of neurodevelopment in children and young adults. *Neuroimage.* 2005;26(4):1164–1173. http://dx.doi.org/10.1016/j.neuroimage.2005.03.016.

13. Thatcher RW. Maturation of the human frontal lobes. Physiological evidence for staging. *Developmental Neuropsychology.* 1991;7(3):397–419.

14. Uematsu A, Matsui M, Tanaka C, et al. Developmental trajectories of amygdala and hippocampus from infancy to early adulthood in healthy individuals. *PLoS One.* 2012;7(10):e46970. http://dx.doi.org/10.1371/journal.pone.0046970.

15. Stamm JM, Bourlas AP, Baugh CM, et al. Age of first exposure to football and later-life cognitive impairment in former NFL players. *Neurology.* 2015;84(11):1114–1120. http://dx.doi.org/10.1212/WNL.0000000000001358.

16. Stamm JM, Koerte IK, Muehlmann M, et al. Age at first exposure to football is associated with altered corpus callosum white matter microstructure in former professional football players. *Journal of Neurotrauma.* 2015;32(22):1768–1776. http://dx.doi.org/10.1089/neu.2014.3822.

17. Montenigro PH, Alosco ML, Martin BM, et al. Cumulative head impact exposure predicts later-life depression, apathy, executive dysfunction, and cognitive impairment in former high school and college football players. *Journal of Neurotrauma.* 2016. http://dx.doi.org/10.1089/neu.2016.4413.

18. Radloff LS. The CES-D scale: a self-report depression scale for research in the general population. *Applied Psychological Measurement.* 1977;1:385–401.

19. Gavett BE, Crane PK, Dams-O'Connor K. Bi-factor analyses of the Brief Test of Adult Cognition by Telephone. *NeuroRehabilitation.* 2013;32:253–265.

20. Roth RM, Isquith PK, Gioia GA. *BRIEF-A: Behavior Rating Inventory of Executive Function-Adult Version: Professional Manual.* Lutz, FL: Psychological Assessment Resources; 2005.

21. McKee AC, Cairns NJ, Dickson DW, et al. The first NINDS/NIBIB consensus meeting to define neuropathological criteria for the diagnosis of chronic traumatic encephalopathy. *Acta Neuropathologica.* 2016;131(1):75–86. http://dx.doi.org/10.1007/s00401-015-1515-z.

22. Montenigro PH, Baugh CM, Daneshvar DH, et al. Clinical subtypes of chronic traumatic encephalopathy: literature review and proposed research diagnostic criteria for traumatic encephalopathy syndrome. *Alzheimer's Research and Therapy.* 2014;6(5):68. http://dx.doi.org/10.1186/s13195-014-0068-z.

23. Stern RA, Daneshvar DH, Baugh CM, et al. Clinical presentation of chronic traumatic encephalopathy. *Neurology.* 2013;81(13):1122–1129. http://dx.doi.org/10.1212/WNL.0b013e3182a55f7f.

24. Alosco ML, Jarnagin J, Tripodis Y, et al. Olfactory function and associated clinical correlates in former national football league players. *Journal of Neurotrauma.* 2016. http://dx.doi.org/10.1089/neu.2016.4536.

25. Alosco ML, Tripodis Y, Jarnagin J, et al. Repetitive head impact exposure and later-life plasma total tau in former NFL players. *Alzheimer's & Dementia: Diagnosis, Assessment & Disease Monitoring.* 2017;7:33–40.

26. Koerte IK, Hufschmidt J, Muehlmann M, et al. Cavum septi pellucidi in symptomatic former professional football players. *Journal of Neurotrauma.* 2016;33(4):346–353. http://dx.doi.org/10.1089/neu.2015.3880.

27. Stern RA, Tripodis Y, Baugh CM, et al. Preliminary study of plasma exosomal tau as a potential biomarker for chronic traumatic encephalopathy. *Journal of Alzheimer's Disease.* 2016;51(4):1099–1109. http://dx.doi.org/10.3233/jad-151028.

CHAPTER 4

Biomechanics of Head Trauma

STEVEN ROWSON • BETHANY ROWSON

INTRODUCTION

I come from a different background than most of the other speakers here. I am an engineer that focuses on injury biomechanics, which is the study of the mechanical input to the human body that causes injury. If we understand those biomechanical forces, we can design protective equipment to prevent injury from occurring. What I hope to accomplish with this talk is to provide an overview of the history of head injury biomechanics that will explain the basis of automotive and sports protective equipment safety standards. I will then discuss more recent work regarding what we know about concussions today, as well as the future directions of concussion biomechanics research.

ACCELERATION-BASED BRAIN INJURY

To start, I want to introduce the concept of acceleration-based brain injury. Acceleration is the rate of change in velocity. For example, you could be in a car going 30 mph and slowly brake for a stop sign, changing your velocity from 30 to 0 mph without any injuries. The 30-mph velocity change is over a relatively long duration, resulting in a low acceleration. On the other hand, you could also be traveling at 30 mph and hit a wall, going from 30 to 0 mph in a very short time period and resulting in a higher acceleration for the same change in velocity. You are more likely to experience injury with the high acceleration case. This general concept also applies to the brain. Since the brain is not rigidly attached to the skull, you get some relative motion between the two. When your head is accelerated, it creates inertial loading on the brain, which could be from direct head impact or an indirect force transmitted through the neck. In injury biomechanics, we typically use acceleration because we can easily measure it to characterize injury risk. It is important to keep in mind that the acceleration of the skull is not what is causing injury, but rather injury results from the pressure and strain responses in the brain associated with acceleration of the skull, as Dr. Robert Cantu discussed in Chapter 1. However, if we understand biomechanically what is happening to the skull, we have a pretty good idea of what is happening to the brain. Acceleration of the skull consists of two components: linear acceleration and rotational acceleration. Linear acceleration of the skull produces a transient pressure gradient within the brain tissue. Rotational acceleration creates relative motion between the brain and skull. This relative motion results in various types of strains within the tissue, which is likely the true injury mechanism of concussion.

The relationships between skull acceleration and brain motion have been experimentally verified. A study from 2007 used cadaver heads with neutral density targets implanted in the brain.[1] These targets were the same density as the brain so that they would not move relative to the tissue and were radiopaque, allowing motion to be tracked during impact with high-speed radiography. The heads were impacted at varying levels of severity, with and without a helmet. They looked at the response of the brain during these impacts and found that it does not "flop" around in the skull as some suggest. You are really getting about 5 to 7 mm of motion relative to the skull, which follows a looping figure eight pattern as the brain rebounds. They also found that head kinematics was related to the pressure response and motion pattern of the brain. Pressure was correlated to the pressure response, and rotational kinematics was related to the brain motion. Acceleration isn't the whole story, as duration also plays an important role. The longer you experience an acceleration, the less tolerable it becomes. If your head experiences an acceleration of $100g$ for 1 ms, you are much less likely to be injured than if it experienced $100g$ for 20 ms. I want you to keep these fundamental principles in mind while I present the historical head injury biomechanics research.

Studying brain injury biomechanics is challenging because we can't ask people to come into the lab and hit their heads to see what happens. Additionally, brain injuries are typically associated with a physiologic response that can't be reproduced with a cadaver. So, we need experimental models that characterize injury in indirect ways. Some early animal model work was done with dogs and then primates, but most current models use rodents or pigs. Although these are all valuable, they still aren't human and certain assumptions need to be made to translate the injurious biomechanical parameters to humans.

WAYNE STATE TOLERANCE CURVE

In 1954, Ford funded research at Wayne State University to determine human tolerance to head injury in order to improve motor vehicle safety. This work focused on skull fracture and pressure gradients inside the brain resulting from direct blows to the head, while measuring head acceleration to correlate to injury risk. Skull fracture was used as the injury outcome based on the clinical observation that concussion was present in 80% of patients with a simple linear skull fracture. The definition of concussion used here was more severe than what we think of today, with all patients presenting with a loss of consciousness. These studies involved an indirect measure of concussion by using an easily observed end point in their experimental model. In 1960, Lissner and colleagues published a study as part of these efforts that involved dropping cadaver heads on plates, floors, and different padded surfaces with a single accelerometer on the back of the skull.[2] From a handful of these tests, they picked out six data points to create the very first head injury tolerance curve, which later became known as the Wayne State Tolerance Curve (WSTC). The curve represents tolerance for skull fracture to impacts 1 to 6 ms in duration, so if you experience accelerations above it, you would likely be injured. What's interesting about this curve is that it is more or less the basis of every existing head injury standard that's in play today, and it's based on six data points from tests in the 1950s. It's amazing how useful these six data points are and how well they have prevented deaths from head injuries.

In 1961, Gurdjian extended the WSTC out to 10 ms in duration, based on animal data using air pressure pulses on exposed dura to induce concussion.[2–4] The intracranial pressure and clinical outcome from animal tests were related to injurious head accelerations in humans through cadaver impacts in which both intracranial pressure and acceleration were measured.[2,4] Although there were no human injury data around this time, some volunteer data were available. John Stapp is well known for his work in injury biomechanics, and he was a volunteer in his own experiments, exposing himself to high-acceleration events on a sled. His tests went up to around $42g$ without any injury, so that was

the original asymptote that extended the curve from 10 to 100 ms.[5,6] With additional volunteer data, the curve's asymptote was updated to $80g$ as an expected tolerance for padded impacts.[5,6] The final version of the WSTC is presented in Fig. 4.1. Again, if an impact's acceleration and duration fall above this curve, you exceed the tolerance level and are likely to sustain injury, while if they fall below the curve, you are not likely to sustain injury. The WSTC has been criticized since its development because it is based on just a few data points from experiments performed in the 1950s and 1960s. There is poor documentation of those experiments and you need to read a lot of old papers to piece it together, and even then there are still holes in it. The definition of acceleration used throughout development of the curve varied; sometimes it referred to average acceleration, sometimes peak acceleration. Despite these criticisms, the WSTC became the basis of all existing head injury standards, from cars to football helmets to bicycle helmets—any form of head protection.

Two injury metrics were developed from the WSTC because it cannot be directly implemented in practice. The curve was drawn based on available data, and was not a mathematical function. The Severity Index (SI) was developed as a linear approximation of the tolerance curve on the log-log scale, resulting in a model of the curve that could be implemented practically. In 1973, the National Operating Committee on Standards for Athletic Equipment (NOCSAE) implemented an SI threshold of 1500 for a football helmet standard based on recommendations from Gadd, who developed SI.[5,7] That had immediate effects, with an approximate 50% reduction in fatal head injuries after the standard was implemented.[5,7] Shortly after that, Ford developed another metric as a mathematical model of the WSTC known as the Head Injury Criterion (HIC).[8] Although the merits of each metric were argued, it turned out they both produced similar results since they were both weighted functions of linear acceleration magnitude and duration. The automotive industry chose to use HIC and eventually they settled at a tolerance threshold of 1000. Both football helmet and automotive standard thresholds were later reduced upon further analysis of the original WSTC impacts. In regards to head injury safety standards, the automotive industry and sports helmets are in agreement. The injury metrics are inherently similar since they are trying to model the same thing. Both weight acceleration magnitude so that it is more important than impact duration, although they both contribute to injury risk. Even with the limitations of the WSTC, safety standards developed from it are very effective at preventing fatal and catastrophic head

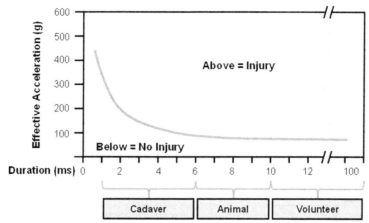

FIG. 4.1 Final iteration of the Wayne State Tolerance Curve. The *line* represents human tolerance to head acceleration and shows that tolerable accelerations decrease with increasing pulse duration. Above the curve, injury is likely, whereas below it, injury is less likely. This curve was developed from multiple datasets using cadaver heads, animal models, and human volunteers for noninjurious accelerations. The cadaver heads were dropped onto rigid surfaces with the tolerance curve line representing skull fracture, which was thought to be representative of a moderate to severe concussion. For the animal models, air pressure pulses were applied directly to the dural surface in dogs for a similar concussive effect. The animal tests were related to humans through intracranial pressure measurements and additional cadaver tests. The asymptote of the curve was estimated based on accelerations that human volunteers experienced during sled tests without any injury.

injuries. The motor vehicle fatality rate has continued to decrease since these standards were implemented. The NOCSAE standard has essentially eliminated acute, catastrophic brain injury in football; there are maybe one or two each year, but considering the number of people playing football the rates are essentially zero.

So why are these standards so effective if the data they are based on are limited? It's essentially because they were the first attempts to limit energy input to the head. Before these standards were put into place, there was no regulation, and it turned out that the thresholds were a pretty good approximation of what causes injury. It's important to note that we are not evaluating the mechanism of brain injury with these standards, but rather a correlate to catastrophic head injury. We do this because it's convenient to measure. We can use a crash test dummy in the lab with accelerometers and measure the head impact response for different events and use that correlate to determine whether there would be an injury or not.

BRAIN INJURY BIOMECHANICS

I am now going to transition to the biomechanics associated with mechanisms that result in injury. We are going to talk about rotation-based brain injury,

which will take us a little further back in time to 1943. Because of the incompressible nature of brain tissue, Holbourn proposed a theory in which translation (or linear motion) would be harmless and only rotation could initiate the strains that are required to produce concussive injuries.[9,10] He used an experimental model that was a section of brain made out of gelatin with a rotational jerk applied and identified where the strains were in the brain during the applied load. His theory resulted in a large body of research evaluating the contributions of linear and rotational acceleration to brain injury. From 1960 to 1980 there were six major datasets that involved both impact and nonimpact tests on primates. Ommaya and Gennarelli were the main contributors to these data, which were very unique and couldn't be collected today. However, these data are often cited as to why only rotational acceleration matters for diffuse brain injuries. Rotation is an important component, but it's not the whole story, which I will demonstrate by looking at a few of these studies. Ommaya and Gennarelli developed a head injury paradigm (Fig. 4.2).[11] Looking at this paradigm, the input to the head can be either static or dynamic, with static being a slow crushing injury and dynamic being what we are interested in relation to concussions. For concussive injuries, the dynamic response of the head can

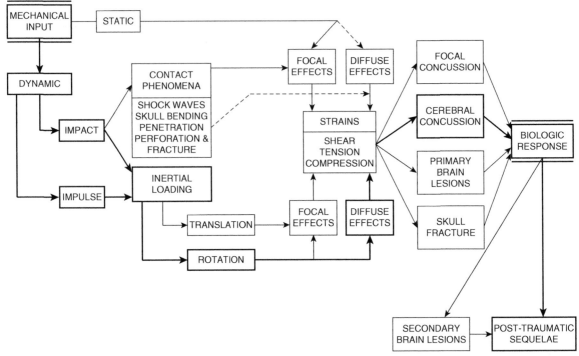

FIG. 4.2 Head injury paradigm developed by Ommaya and Gennarelli. The paradigm explains the basic mechanisms and injuries thought to result from different mechanical inputs. Although different mechanisms are involved depending on the input, strains within the brain ultimately lead to clinical signs and pathology. (With permission from Ommaya AK. Biomechanics of Head Injuries: Experimental Aspects. In: Melvin ANaJW, ed. *Biomechanics of Trauma*. East Norwalk, CT: Appleton-Century-Crofts; 1985.)

result either from an impact (a blow to the head) or an impulse transmitted through the body without impact to the head. An impact results in both inertial loading of the head and contact effects, meaning skull deformation, causing a pressure response and focal injuries (like contusions) in the brain. Different types of blows and different scenarios result in translation and rotation of the head, with translation being associated with focal affects, while rotation can contribute to focal and diffuse effects. Essentially, this causes stretching of the brain tissue that results in an injury response. Ommaya and Gennarelli wanted to experimentally verify this paradigm, so they performed a number of experiments that evaluated the contributions of linear and rotational acceleration to brain injury and the differences in observed injuries between impact and inertial loads. I will go through a few studies now that highlight those two questions: linear versus rotational acceleration and impact versus inertial or nonimpact.

An inertial loading apparatus was developed that eliminated head contact, in which the primate subject wore a helmet fixed to the skull that was attached to an acceleration device.[11-13] The primate's head could be moved to induce translation only or a combination of translation and rotation by moving the head in an arc, with a pivot point in the cervical spine (Fig. 4.3). They looked at the injury response with different accelerative inputs of pure translation ranging from around 700g to 1200g and tangential acceleration in the rotational cases ranging from 300g to 1000g. So both modes had similar inputs in terms of linear acceleration, but for the translation only cases, they did not see concussion, while the rotation cases produced concussion with distinct injury patterns. There were focal effects for the translation only group in about half of the animals, while there were much more diffuse injuries in nearly all of the rotated animals. So pure translation did not produce diffuse damage, it was only when rotation was added to translation that diffuse injuries were seen. There was not a rotation only event here since the head pivoted about a point in the neck, with that pivot point being the only point to not experience linear acceleration.

TRANSLATION   ROTATION

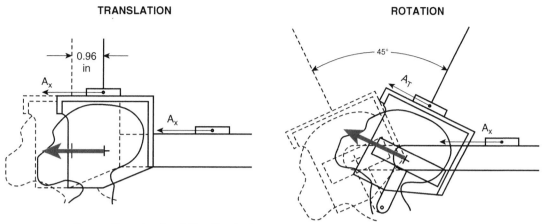

FIG. 4.3 Gennarelli used an inertial loading device to determine the relative dependence of translational and rotational motion in brain injuries in a controlled manner without direct impact. The device included a helmet molded to a primate subject's head to distribute the load and eliminate focal effects. The device could accelerate the head in a translation-only motion (left) or pivot about a point in the neck for a combination of translational and rotational motion. (With permission from Ommaya AK. Biomechanics of Head Injuries: Experimental Aspects. In: Melvin ANaJW, ed. *Biomechanics of Trauma*. East Norwalk, CT: Appleton-Century-Crofts; 1985.)

Holbourn's theory also implied that since rotation is a critical mechanism, injury shouldn't depend on how the rotation is initiated. If this was true, injury would occur at a particular rotational velocity, regardless of whether it occurred as a result of an impact to the head or an impulse transmitted to the head. The difference is that the impact would be at a higher acceleration, similar to the analogy of a car slowly stopping versus hitting a wall. Ommaya's experiments evaluated this aspect of Holbourn's theory by comparing whiplash-type injuries without head impact to direct head impacts in primates.[14-16] The data showed that twice the rotational velocity was needed to produce concussion for indirect impacts compared to direct impacts, implying that the contact phenomenon plays a role. The summation of rotational and translational effects contributes to injury, and the acceleration is higher for impact events versus impulse, lowering the rotational velocity threshold.

One last study I'll go over was done by Gennarelli in 1982, showing a directional dependence in head injury thresholds using another nonimpact accelerative device with primates.[17,18] So for the same input acceleration to the head, the injury outcome varied depending on the direction on loading. In general, for the same input to the head, coronal rotation produced more injury than sagittal rotation.

Animal data are great for fundamental research, and we have learned a lot from these studies, but they are limited in application to humans because the brains in animal models are different in size, anatomy, and geometry from humans. So when we want to use primate data to determine what human head injury tolerance should be, we have to scale it. There are different physical laws we can follow to compare masses between species and get an idea of what a human would experience relative to a primate to cause the same injury. These laws assume the geometry and material properties of the brain are the same between species, only accounting for differences in mass. So you need to transform the data in some way and there are a lot of errors introduced in doing that, but it gives us a good ballpark estimate. Ommaya scaled his primate data to humans in terms of rotational velocities and accelerations (Fig. 4.4).[19,20] What these data show is that velocity and acceleration are both important to injury outcome. You want to consider velocity because it gives an indication of how long acceleration levels are experienced. We can use a woodpecker as an extreme example of scaling. A human has a brain mass of 1400 g while a woodpecker has a brain mass of 2 g. Even a 1000g impact in a woodpecker would only be around 100g in a human based on mass scaling. There are a lot of other factors there, but brain mass plays an important role in injury tolerance because the more massive the brain is, the more inertia it has, which in turn will create more strains within itself.

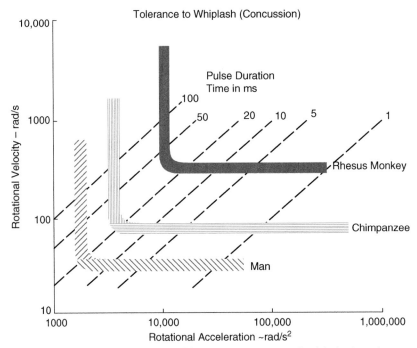

FIG. 4.4 Scaling relationships were determined for noncontact concussion injuries based on experimental data from different-sized primates. The injury thresholds in terms of rotational velocity and acceleration were scaled to human based on average brain mass for the species. Injury severity was thought to be more closely related to rotational velocity for short-duration impacts, whereas rotational acceleration was thought to be more relevant for longer durations. (With permission from Ommaya AK. Biomechanics of Head Injuries: Experimental Aspects. In: Melvin ANaJW, ed. *Biomechanics of Trauma*. East Norwalk, CT: Appleton-Century-Crofts; 1985.)

CONCUSSIVE IMPACTS IN FOOTBALL

Transitioning now to more modern concussion work, we'll start out with a study looking at reconstructions of concussive impacts in National Football League (NFL) players. In this study, they looked at concussive events on film that had multiple camera angles and used the difference between position and pixel space between two cameras to triangulate a three-dimensional (3D) position for the players involved in the impact.[21] Essentially, they can determine the 3D position of players in each frame of video and get impact velocities that can then be used to recreate these scenarios in the lab with dummies. The dummies are instrumented with accelerometers to get the head accelerations associated with these impacts that players experience, so they are matching dummy impacts with game film. They reconstructed 25 concussions and saw that the average concussion occurred around 100g and 6500 rad/s². This is a really neat dataset because they are quantifying the input for a more current definition of concussion

in terms of biomechanics. The study was limited by a small sample size and nearly equal numbers of injury and noninjury data points. In reality, there are many nonconcussive head impacts for every concussive one, so you can't quantify injury risk from these data.

Around the same time as the NFL study in 2003, researchers were starting to look at football players as a unique opportunity to collect biomechanical data that could characterize injury. These players hit their heads willingly on a regular basis, so you can instrument and observe this population that is at an elevated risk of injury. In 2003 at Virginia Tech, we started measuring head acceleration in Virginia Tech football players with instrumentation inside their helmets.[22] The instrumentation consists of six accelerometers that are spring mounted so that they stay in contact with the head and measure head acceleration, rather than helmet acceleration. Data are collected for every practice and game, so any time players experience accelerations over 10g, we collect a 40-ms window of acceleration

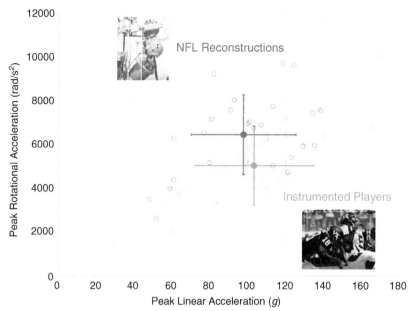

FIG. 4.5 Linear and rotational accelerations were similar for concussive impacts in football players using two very different methods. The first dataset came from laboratory reconstructions of NFL impacts causing concussion, whereas the second dataset came from instrumented football players sustaining a concussion.[21,23,28,31]

data. These impact durations are generally on the order of 10 ms, so we get a little before and after the impact. Each event is time stamped, and we compare to video to confirm the impact occurred. We've done this for 13 years, and other schools have instrumented their players in the same manner. There are now more than 2 million data points from people using this type of instrumentation in helmets.[22-31] What's especially unique about this dataset is that it's from humans. There are limitations, but you can start to understand the biomechanical input that produces injury. So if we separate impacts that resulted in injury and ones that didn't, you can see that subconcussive impacts average 26g for linear acceleration, about 1000 rad/s² for rotational acceleration, and 5 rad/s for rotational velocity. Our concussive impacts are higher at 105g, 5000 rad/s², and about 22 rad/s.[32,33] These impacts are all very similar in duration, around 8 to 12 ms. When we compare these volunteer helmet data to the NFL reconstruction data, we actually see good agreement between them. The average NFL concussion was $98 \pm 27g$, while the first 32 volunteer concussions were $105 \pm 27g$. The fact that two very different methodologies resulted in similar values is evidence that these numbers are both in the ballpark of acceleration input to the head that causes concussion. The rotational accelerations from

these two datasets were also similar, again suggesting these numbers are in the right ballpark (Fig. 4.5).

We can also compare the football data to some of the thresholds derived from animal models (Fig. 4.6). Ommaya's concussion threshold from scaled primate data falls right within the ranges of both football datasets in terms of rotational acceleration and velocity.[19] Other scaled data from primates and rodents for more severe diffuse axonal injury (DAI) are higher in magnitude than the concussion data, as would be expected for a more severe injury.[34,35] Even though these data were collected in different manners from different species, they further suggest that the average values for concussion are in the right ballpark.

When looking at impact direction, we can divide the volunteer concussive impacts into ones that resulted in sagittal or coronal rotation and then impacts to the top of the head. We see that linear acceleration levels are very similar to one another for all directions, but rotational acceleration is less for top impacts, but still capable of producing injury (Fig. 4.7).[33] We see different relationships between linear and rotational acceleration for impacts to the top of the head versus sagittal or coronal rotation.

We can look at the distributions of acceleration for volunteer impacts resulting in injury and those

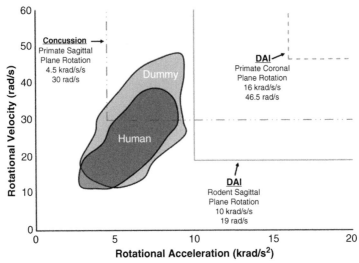

FIG. 4.6 The data from NFL reconstructions (dummy) and instrumented football players (human) can be compared with various thresholds for brain injury scaled from animal models.[21,23,28,31] The scaled concussion threshold from primate experiments falls right within the human concussion data, whereas scaled thresholds for much more severe injuries (diffuse axonal injury) are generally greater than the concussive values.[19,34,35]

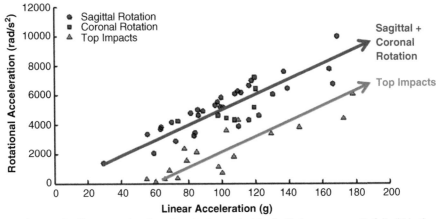

FIG. 4.7 Concussive linear accelerations from instrumented football players generally fall within the same range regardless of impact location, but rotational accelerations vary for impacts to the top of the head. Top impacts tend to have lower rotational accelerations for similar linear accelerations while still causing injury. (With permission from Rowson S, et al. Rotational head kinematics in football impacts: an injury risk function for concussion. *Annals of Biomedical Engineering.* 2012;40(1):1–13.)

not resulting in injury separately. For both linear and rotational accelerations, the concussive impacts are normally distributed, while the subconcussive impacts are right-skewed (Fig. 4.8).[32,33] The most interesting aspect of these distributions is the region of overlap between them, which describes where risk changes for individuals. For values within that region of overlap,

there is a subset of the population who will get injured and another subset who won't. We can quantify injury risk based on these data. We have done that for linear and rotational accelerations separately, and you can see that risk is very low and changes very little until around 100g and 4000 rad/s².[32,33] We also know that every head impact has a combination of linear and

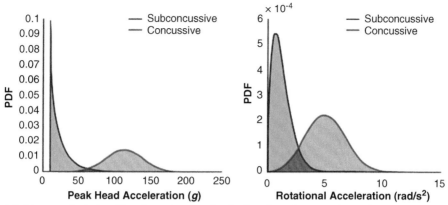

FIG. 4.8 Linear and rotational head acceleration distributions for subconcussive and concussive impacts in instrumented football players.[33,42] It can be seen that the subconcussive impacts are right-skewed and lower than the concussive impacts, whereas the concussive impacts have normal distributions. The region of overlap between subconcussive and concussive distributions is where the risk of injury changes. *PDF*, probability density function.

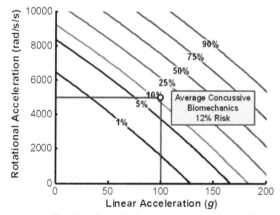

FIG. 4.9 The bivariate risk function is dependent on linear and rotational head accelerations and was developed from instrumented football player data.[36] The function is represented as a contour plot here, so each *line* represents a constant risk value for different combinations of linear and rotational accelerations. The average concussive linear and rotational accelerations are only associated with approximately 12% risk of injury, because most of the impacts at this level do not result in injury.

rotational accelerations; it's never just one or the other. It doesn't make a lot of sense to analyze them independently, so more recently we developed a bivariate risk function that includes both (Fig. 4.9).[36] If we look at the average concussion around 100g and 5000 rad/s², the risk function estimates a 12% probability of injury. That means about one in every eight people might get hurt if they experience that impact. I am talking about

risk, but people often talk about injuries in terms of thresholds, so I'll go through a hypothetical situation to clarify what that means. If we have a linear acceleration threshold of 150g, that implies that all accelerations below 150g won't result in injury, while all accelerations above 150g would. But we know that risk is continuous over that range, and there is not some magic threshold where everyone will or will not be hurt. Whenever you pick a threshold, you are actually picking a specified risk value, or defining an acceptable level of risk.

CONCUSSIVE IMPACTS IN YOUNGER AGES

There are 5 million football players in the United States, and the majority of these players are between 6 and 13 years old (Fig. 4.10). However, most research to date has focused on high school through NFL players rather than the adolescent level. There is reason to think that concussion tolerance would change as a function of age and gender, so how do we understand that? We recently started a new study in which we are investigating head impact exposure in youth football. Specifically, what is the exposure to head impact that these players experience and do we see variations in clinical data based on this exposure? For biomechanical data, we are looking at linear and rotational head accelerations, impact frequency, and impact location. For clinical data, we are collecting sign and symptom assessments, cognitive tests using the NIH tool box, and balance assessments. All clinical data are collected preseason, during the season if an injury occurs, and postseason. These

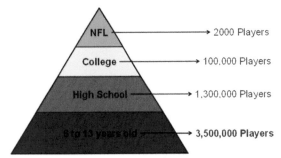

FIG. 4.10 Although most head injury research to date has focused on high school through professional athletes, the majority of football players are at the youth level. It is likely that concussion tolerance changes as a function of age, and the effects of injury on the developing brain are not fully understood. Therefore, more data are needed to determine concussion biomechanics for youth athletes.

measurements are then correlated with biomechanical data. We have collected data on 324 youth football players between 7 and 14 years old, resulting in more than 15,000 head impacts.[37–41] Head impact exposure varies by age for two main reasons: the number of practices and games increases with age, and player athleticism and aggressiveness increase with age. These factors also increase the severity of impacts that occur. We have also captured a few concussions from these youth players, with average linear acceleration of $61 \pm 28g$ and average rotational acceleration of 3020 ± 1230 rad/ s^2.[37] These values are lower than the collective values measured for 105 adult concussions across many studies, with averages of $102 \pm 34g$ and 3977 ± 2272 rad/s^2. However, there exists a much larger sample (105) of adult concussions compared to a small sample (4) of youth concussions. More data are needed to determine how concussion tolerance changes with age.

TOWARD REDUCING CONCUSSIVE IMPACTS IN ATHLETES

Although we still need more data before fully understanding how head injury tolerance changes with age, we can implement strategies now that reduce concussions in these athletes. If we reduce the number of times players hit their heads, we reduce exposure to impact and therefore risk of injury. Rule changes and teaching proper techniques to athletes will reduce their head impact exposure. As an example of these changes to reduce exposure, when looking at our youth football data, we saw that the majority of high head accelerations experienced were associated with a specific drill where players ran at each other head on.[38]

We published those data and made recommendations based on it, and Pop Warner subsequently instituted new rules to reduce contact in practice. In the second year of that study, we compared teams who adopted the new rules to those who didn't and saw a 50% reduction in head impact exposure from limiting contact in practice.[37] That's just one example of how data-driven decisions can be made to reduce head impact exposure for players.

Since we can't eliminate all head impacts from sports, it is important to have good protective headgear to reduce the severity of the impacts that do occur. Helmets play an important role in managing energy input into the head during an impact. The two primary components to any helmet are the shell and the liner (or padding). The role of the shell is to deflect and distribute force over a larger area, while the liner modulates how that energy is transferred to the head. The foam reduces acceleration magnitude by extending duration. As I mentioned earlier, it is more important to reduce magnitude than it is to reduce duration, although they both contribute to injury risk. The helmet manages the way energy is transferred to the head, and you can design a helmet in such a way to optimally reduce head acceleration magnitude.

After we had been instrumenting our football players for a number of years, our equipment manager at Virginia Tech was looking to buy new helmets and asked us what he should buy. We bought a few and started testing them in the lab, and we saw there were big differences in head accelerations for identical impacts between helmet types. These were all helmets that passed the NOCSAE safety standard, but some were just under the threshold while others were well under it. These differences in acceleration produce differences in concussion risk for the same impact. For example, comparing one of the best performing helmets to the worst helmet for an identical impact to the crown of the helmet, the better helmet resulted in a head acceleration of $84g$, while the worst performing resulted in $190g$. That's over a 50% reduction in head acceleration between helmet models, which relates to a huge difference in concussion risk.

After seeing how differently the available helmets performed, we started the Virginia Tech Helmet Ratings (www.vt.edu/helmet) to evaluate different types of head protection in an effort to inform consumers.[42,43] We currently rate football and hockey helmets but are expanding to bicycle helmets and soccer headgear, as well as other areas including commercial head impact sensors. Our helmet evaluations are based on two fundamental principles: (1) each test we do in the lab is weighted based on how frequently a similar impact would occur on the field, and (2) helmets that lower acceleration reduce risk of concussion. We know how frequently each type of lab impact occurs on the field from years of data from instrumented athletes. We quantify risk for each impact in the lab and then multiply that by exposure and predict incidence of injury. We see a range of acceleration values for different helmet types, and we assign a number of stars based on the cumulative risk associated with each helmet. We make that data available to the public so that consumers can make informed decisions and manufacturers can make improvements to their designs. In 2011 when we released the first football helmet ratings, there was only one five-star helmet, now there are 16 football helmets that earn five stars.

Predicted injury incidence results from laboratory-based football helmet evaluations were confirmed on the field.[42,44] We tracked players and which helmets they wore from eight different universities that instrumented their football players during the same 5-year period. The neat thing about this study was that since all players had instrumentation in their helmets, we could control for the number of head impacts each experienced in each type of helmet. That way you aren't comparing a player in a bad helmet who never plays, and therefore has a low risk of injury, to a player in a better performing helmet with higher head impact exposure. We saw that the laboratory prediction of difference in the concussion rate was right around the same range that we saw on the field. These on-field data demonstrate that helmets that reduce head acceleration reduce risk of concussion. Helmets won't eliminate injury, but if you reduce risk and have millions people of playing football, it's going to reduce injury incidence and rate.

Last year, we started rating hockey helmets using methods that included linear and rotational accelerations, and they performed a whole lot worse than football helmets.[43] We were curious how the thickness of the padding in their helmets compared to what they wear on the rest of their body since the helmets didn't perform very well and saw that the thinnest padding is what they wear to protect their heads. If we compare the padding thickness between football and hockey helmets, the hockey helmet has about half the padding, meaning hockey helmets can't manage energy as well as football helmets can.

Can all concussions be prevented? No, any player in any sport can sustain a head injury. There are many factors contributing to injury risk like genetics, individual tolerance, and neck strength. Helmets also don't cover the entire head, so they can only protect what they cover. Until more advanced materials are designed,

helmets are limited by size and padding thickness. Not all concussions can be prevented, but risk can be minimized, and even small reductions in risk over a very large number of people can result in substantial reductions in the number of injuries.

REFERENCES

1. Hardy WN, et al. A study of the response of the human cadaver head to impact. *The Stapp Car Crash Journal.* 2007;51:17–80.
2. Lissner HR, Lebow M, Evans FG. Experimental studies on the relation between acceleration and intracranial pressure changes in man. *Surgery, Gynecology & Obstetrics.* 1960;111:329–338.
3. Gurdijan ES, Webster JE, Lissner HR. Observations on the mechanism of brain concussion, contusion, and laceration. Surgery. *Gynecology and Obstetrics.* 1955;101:680–690.
4. Gurdjian E, et al. Intracranial pressure and acceleration accompanying head impacts in human cadavers. *Surgery Gynecology & Obstetrics.* 1961;113:185.
5. SAE. Human tolerance to impact conditions as related to motor vehicle design – SAE J885. In: *SAE Information Report.* 1986.
6. Patrick LM, Lissner HR, Gurdijan ES. Survival by design – head protection. In: *Proceedings of the 7th Stapp Car Crash Conference.* 1963:483–499.
7. Mertz HJ, Prasad P, Nusholtz G. Head injury risk assessment for forehead impacts. In: *International Congress and Exposition.* 1996. Detroit, MI: SAE Paper No. 960099.
8. Versace J. A review of the severity index. *SAE Technical Paper Series.* 1971. SAE 710881.
9. Holbourn AHS. Mechanics of head injuries. *Lancet.* 1943;2:438–441.
10. Holbourn AHS. The mechanics of brain injuries. *British Medical Bulletin.* 1945;3(6):147–149.
11. Ommaya AK, Gennarelli TA. Cerebral concussion and traumatic unconsciousness. Correlation of experimental and clinical observations of blunt head injuries. *Brain.* 1974;97(4):633–654.
12. Gennarelli T, Ommaya A, Thibault L. Comparison of translational and rotational head motions in experimental cerebral concussion. In: *Proc. 15th Stapp Car Crash Conference.* 1971.
13. Gennarelli TA, Thibault LE, Ommaya AK. Pathophysiologic responses to rotational and translational accelerations of the head. *SAE Technical Paper Series.* 1972:296–308. 720970.
14. Ommaya A, Corrao P. Pathologic biomechanics of central nervous system injury in head impact and whiplash trauma. In: *Proceedings of the international conference on accident pathology.* Washington, DC: Government Printing Office; 1970.
15. Ommaya AK, Faas F, Yarnell P. Whiplash injury and brain damage: an experimental study. *JAMA.* 1968;204(4):285–289.

16. Ommaya AK, Hirsch AE, Martinez JL. The role of whiplash in cerebral concussion. In: *Proc. 10th Stapp Car Crash Conference*. 1966.

17. Gennarelli TA, et al. Diffuse axonal injury and traumatic coma in the primate. *Annals of Neurology*. 1982;12(6):564–574.

18. Gennarelli T, et al. Directional dependence of axonal brain injury due to centroidal and non-centroidal acceleration. *SAE Technical Paper Series*. 1987:49–53. 872197.

19. Ommaya AK. Biomechanics of Head Injuries: experimental Aspects. In: Melvin ANaJW, ed. *Biomechanics of Trauma*. Eat Norwalk, CT: Appleton-Century-Crofts; 1985.

20. Ommaya AK, et al. Scaling of experimental data on cerebral concussion in sub-human primates to concussion threshold for man. In: *Proceedings of the 11th Stapp Car Crash Conference*. 1967. SAE 670906.

21. Pellman EJ, et al. Concussion in professional football: reconstruction of game impacts and injuries. *Neurosurgery*. 2003;53(4):799–812. Discussion 812-4.

22. Duma SM, et al. Analysis of real-time head accelerations in collegiate football players. *Clinical Journal of Sport Medicine*. 2005;15(1):3–8.

23. Broglio SP, et al. Biomechanical properties of concussions in high school football. *Medicine & Science in Sports & Exercise*. 2010;42(11):2064–2071.

24. Crisco JJ, et al. Frequency and location of head impact exposures in individual collegiate football players. *Journal of Athletic Training*. 2010;45(6):549–559.

25. Crisco JJ, et al. Head impact exposure in collegiate football players. *Journal of Biomechanics*. 2011;44(15):2673–2678.

26. Crisco JJ, et al. Magnitude of head impact exposures in individual collegiate football players. *Journal of Applied Biomechanics*. 2012;28(2):174–183.

27. Funk JR, et al. Biomechanical risk estimates for mild traumatic brain injury. *Annual Proceedings of the Association for the Advancement of Automotive Medicine*. 2007;51:343–361.

28. Guskiewicz KM, et al. Measurement of head impacts in collegiate football players: relationship between head impact biomechanics and acute clinical outcome after concussion. *Neurosurgery*. 2007;61(6):1244–1253.

29. Mihalik JP, et al. Measurement of head impacts in collegiate football players: an investigation of positional and event-type differences. *Neurosurgery*. 2007;61(6):1229–1235. Discussion 1235.

30. Schnebel B, et al. In vivo study of head impacts in football: a comparison of National Collegiate Athletic Association Division I versus high school impacts. *Neurosurgery*. 2007;60(3):490–495. Discussion 495-6.

31. Duma SM, Rowson S. Every newton hertz: a macro to micro approach to investigating brain injury. *Conference proceedings: … Annual International Conference of the IEEE Engineering in Medicine and Biology Society. IEEE Engineering in Medicine and Biology Society*. 2009;1:1123–1126.

32. Rowson S, Duma SM. *Virginia Tech Helmet Ratings – Adult Football Helmet Ratings*; May 2014. Available from: http://www.sbes.vt.edu/helmet.

33. Rowson S, et al. Rotational head kinematics in football impacts: an injury risk function for concussion. *Annals of Biomedical Engineering*. 2012;40(1):1–13.

34. Davidsson J, Angeria M, Risling MG. Injury threshold for sagittal plane rotational induced diffuse axonal injuries. In: *Proceedings of the International Research Conference on the Biomechanics of Impact (IRCOBI)*. 2009. York, UK.

35. Margulies SS, Thibault LE. A proposed tolerance criterion for diffuse axonal injury in man. *Journal of Biomechanics*. 1992;25(8):917–923.

36. Rowson S, Duma SM. Brain injury prediction: assessing the combined probability of concussion using linear and rotational head acceleration. *Annals of Biomedical Engineering*. 2013;41(5):873–882.

37. Cobb BR, et al. Head impact exposure in youth football: elementary school ages 9–12 years and the effect of practice structure. *Annals of Biomedical Engineering*. 2013a;41(12):2463–2473.

38. Daniel RW, Rowson S, Duma SM. Head impact exposure in youth football. *Annals of Biomedical Engineering*. 2012;40(4):976–981.

39. Daniel RW, Rowson S, Duma SM. Head acceleration measurements in middle school football. *Biomedical Sciences Instrumentation*. 2013;50:291–296.

40. Cobb BR, Rowson S, Duma SM. Age-related differences in head impact exposure of 9–13 year old football players. *Biomedical Sciences Instrumentation*. 2013b;50:285–290.

41. Young T, Rowson S, Duma SM. High magnitude head impacts experienced during youth football practices. *Biomedical Sciences Instrumentation*. 2013;50:100–105.

42. Rowson S, Duma SM. Development of the STAR evaluation system for football helmets: integrating player head impact exposure and risk of concussion. *Annals of Biomedical Engineering*. 2011;39(8):2130–2140.

43. Rowson B, Rowson S, Duma SM. Hockey STAR: a methodology for assessing the biomechanical performance of hockey helmets. *Annals of Biomedical Engineering*. 2015;43(10):2429–2443.

44. Rowson S, et al. Can helmet design reduce the risk of concussion in football? *Journal of Neurosurgery*. 2014;120(4):919–922.

CHAPTER 5

Mechanisms of Concussion, Traumatic Brain Injury, and Chronic Traumatic Encephalopathy: Acute and Chronic Effects of Blast Exposure

LEE GOLDSTEIN

INTRODUCTION

Thank you very much for the nice introduction to the work I am going to present. This work is attempting to relate the pathology that Dr. Ann McKee (Chapter 2) and Dr. Thor Stein (Chapter 8) see in the patients under the microscope to the injuries that cause them. The work that I will be presenting today is from a very large interdisciplinary team in our lab at Boston University (BU), Dr. McKee's lab at the Veterans Affairs (VA) Boston Healthcare System, associated labs affiliated with our Alzheimer's Disease Center, as well as collaborators at Lawrence Livermore National Laboratory, University of Massachusetts, New York Medical College, Harvard University, Ben-Gurion University (Israel), and Oxford University (United Kingdom). We are very grateful for all of our funding and supporters, but especially that from the Concussion Legacy Foundation. We are also grateful to the families and individuals who made this work possible. We sincerely hope that this work will help others in the future.

DEFINITIONS

I want to start with something that is controversial. One of the reasons we are here is because there is a lot of confusion in this field, and part of the confusion is due to definitions. Clarifying these definitions will be helpful scientifically and clinically. *Concussion* is a *neurological syndrome* largely decided by consensus, as discussed by Dr. Robert Cantu (Chapter 1). It's a very dramatic syndrome, but it's a syndrome nonetheless. That means it is a collection of clinical signs and symptoms. *Traumatic brain injury* (TBI) is entirely different. TBI is a *neurological event* and not a disease, just like an acute myocardial infarction (a heart attack) is not a disease in

and of itself. You can have a heart attack as a result of a variety of different causes, and the event itself is the injury. *Chronic traumatic encephalopathy* (CTE) is a *neurological disease*, a tau protein neurodegenerative disorder. Dr. Robert Stern (Chapter 3) mentioned this earlier that we have the *traumatic encephalopathy syndrome*, which is yet again another entity. Keeping these different terms straight is challenging but very important, and we will come back to these definitions and their relation to one another.

One question is whether it is hits or concussions that cause damage or whether we should be monitoring something altogether different, like a biomarker. I am going to tell you it's the latter. We are trying to map these various things, these insults to the injuries, and trying to depict the clinical syndrome when people are still alive. As Dr. McKee and Dr. Stern and others have presented, we have this neurodegenerative disease called CTE, and we would like to know what the relationship is between the injury, the clinical syndrome, and this disease. This relationship is what we need to be focusing on now, as the disease has been very well described by our pathology colleagues, led by Dr. McKee.

Fig. 5.1 shows how in CTE there is a very distinct pattern of atrophy of the brain caused by a tauopathy. There is also a myelinated axonal neuropathy. There is a very unique, distinctive—actually pathognomonic—distribution of tau in the depths of the sulci in and around the microvasculature. So if we think about this disease, we need to be able to explain these features that we see postmortem at the very least. We need to capture these characteristics, and to catch it very early, even in teenagers. I will show you in a moment that, initially, in the early

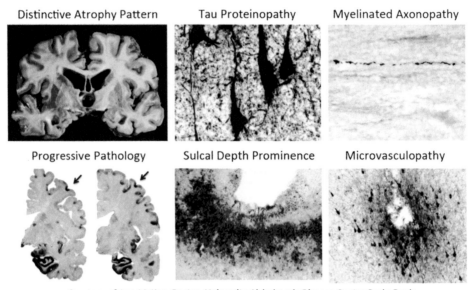

Courtesy of Ann McKee, Boston University Alzheimer's Disease Center Brain Bank

FIG. 5.1 Characteristic pathologic features of chronic traumatic encephalopathy. (Figure courtesy of Dr. Ann McKee, Boston University Alzheimer's Disease Center Brain Bank.)

stages of the disease, CTE involves only regions of the cortex in the depths of the sulci, as well as in and around the vessels. We have to account for the origin of these pathological features if we are to understand the mechanisms that trigger the disease.

CTE IN BLAST AND IMPACT INJURY

I am going to highlight a paper we published a couple years ago that set us on the road to thinking about this problem (Fig. 5.2).[1] As a clinician scientist, I start and finish with the patient—that is the central focus of all this work. The animal work I will present is in the service of understanding this disease in people. Fig. 5.3 shows part of the cortex of a veteran who suffered exposure to a single blast while in military combat. Years later when Dr. McKee looked at his brain we can see the same brown staining of tau pathology that she described in the football players after repetitive impacts. You can see this very interesting pattern of staining here, in and around small blood vessels that are cut in cross-section. What is really striking about this finding is not only the obvious "bullet hole" pattern we see here, but also—and I only realized this after I published this paper—and more importantly, within 100 μm or so from the affected blood vessels, you can see

other vessels that appear not to be affected. This finding would argue that this is not a generalized tissue reaction, but rather there is some sort of focal injury. We saw this pattern in all of the brains in our study, specifically, focal tau pathology around small blood vessels in the depths of the cortical sulci. This is a very important feature of the brain pathology that we need to understand mechanistically. There are clues here to the underlying pathobiology of CTE.

Neuropathological findings are by definition correlative. Neuropathology in these cases cannot establish mechanistic causality. But we can draw some inferences because we have observed that different types of insults are giving rise to similar neuropathology. That is a clue and something we need to pay attention to, because I think we can explain that correlation based on the data I am going to present to you. OK, so we have this pathology, and now we want to ask the question, what is the relationship between the injury and the pathology? Note that we are not necessarily talking about concussion, but rather the injury itself, whether military blast exposure or sports-related head impact. Symptoms possibly related to CTE have been common complaints after military blast exposure dating back to World War I and after sports-related head injuries, especially in boxers, since about the same time.

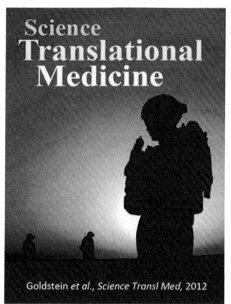

RESEARCH ARTICLE

TRAUMATIC BRAIN INJURY

Chronic Traumatic Encephalopathy in Blast-Exposed Military Veterans and a Blast Neurotrauma Mouse Model

Lee E. Goldstein,[1,2,3,4*] Andrew M. Fisher,[1,4] Chad A. Tagge,[1,4] Xiao-Lei Zhang,[5] Libor Velisek,[5] John A. Sullivan,[5] Chirag Upreti,[5] Jonathan M. Kracht,[4] Maria Ericsson,[6] Mark W. Wojnarowicz,[1] Cezar J. Goletiani,[5] Giorgi M. Maglakelidze,[5] Noel Casey,[1,3] Juliet A. Moncaster,[1,3] Olga Minaeva,[1,3,4] Robert D. Moir,[7] Christopher J. Nowinski,[8] Robert A. Stern,[2,8] Robert C. Cantu,[8,9] James Geiling,[10] Jan K. Blusztajn,[2] Benjamin L. Wolozin,[2] Tsuneya Ikezu,[2] Thor D. Stein,[2,11] Andrew E. Budson,[2,11] Neil W. Kowall,[2,11] David Chargin,[1] Andre Sharon,[4,12] Sudad Saman,[13] Garth F. Hall,[13] William C. Moss,[14] Robin O. Cleveland,[15] Rudolph E. Tanzi,[7] Patric K. Stanton,[5] Ann C. McKee[2,8,11*]

Blast exposure is associated with traumatic brain injury (TBI), neuropsychiatric symptoms, and long-term cognitive disability. We examined a case series of postmortem brains from U.S. military veterans exposed to blast and/or concussive injury. We found evidence of chronic traumatic encephalopathy (CTE), a tau protein–linked neurodegenerative disease, that was similar to the CTE neuropathology observed in young amateur American football players and a professional wrestler with histories of concussive injuries. We developed a blast neurotrauma mouse model that recapitulated CTE-linked neuropathology in wild-type C57BL/6 mice 2 weeks after exposure to a single blast. Blast-exposed mice demonstrated phosphorylated tauopathy, myelinated axonopathy, microvasculopathy, chronic neuroinflammation, and neurodegeneration in the absence of macroscopic tissue damage or hemorrhage. Blast exposure induced persistent hippocampal-dependent learning and memory deficits that persisted for at least 1 month and correlated with impaired axonal conduction and defective activity-dependent long-term potentiation of synaptic transmission. Intracerebral pressure recordings demonstrated that shock waves traversed the mouse brain with minimal change and without thoracic contributions. Kinematic analysis revealed blast-induced head oscillation at accelerations sufficient to cause brain injury. Head immobilization during blast exposure prevented blast-induced learning and memory deficits. The contribution of blast wind to injurious head acceleration may be a primary injury

FIG. 5.2 Chronic traumatic encephalopathy in blast-exposed military veterans and a blast neurotrauma mouse model. (With permission from Goldstein LE, et al. Chronic traumatic encephalopathy in blast-exposed military veterans and a blast neurotrauma mouse model. *Science Translational Medicine.* May 16, 2012;4(134):134ra60.)

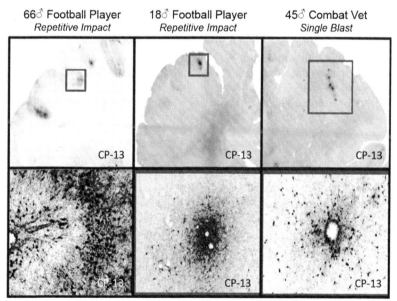

FIG. 5.3 Similar chronic traumatic encephalopathy pathology found in combat veterans exposed to a single blast and football players with repetitive impacts. (With permission from Goldstein LE, et al. Chronic traumatic encephalopathy in blast-exposed military veterans and a blast neurotrauma mouse model. *Science Translational Medicine.* May 16, 2012;4(134):134ra60.)

BLAST NEUROTRAUMA MOUSE MODEL

With our large group of colleagues and collaborators, led out of my laboratory at BU, we have addressed this question of mechanistic causality, the relationship between the traumatic insult involving the head and pathology in the brain. Here we did something a little different. Rather than begin by focusing on scaling the human injury to the animal to see if it would produce the pathology, we started from the reverse. We started by replicating the brain pathology to see if we could work our way back and figure out what characteristics of the injury would be needed to replicate the pathology. The ultimate goal—and Dr. Ramon Diaz-Arrastia (Chapter 12) will speak about this tomorrow—is to facilitate human clinical trials by finding biomarkers and treatments that can then be applied in the clinical setting.

We did this work in collaboration with my colleagues in engineering at BU and with the Lawrence Livermore National Laboratory, which has some of the best blast experts in the world. We developed a new mouse model to replicate what happens in humans (Fig. 5.4). We included high-speed videography at millions of frames per second. This ultrahigh-resolution film record actually makes all the difference, because what I am going to show you happens in fractions of a millisecond. We also allowed the head to move freely, and this is important because we had some indication that it is the head movement that is important, as you just heard from Dr. Steven Rowson (Chapter 4). In this example video, you can see the supersonic blast shock wave move across the screen at 1.35 Mach, that is, 1.35 times faster than the speed of sound. (Video starts.) OK, that's the blast shock wave going by and what you are going to see following it is the moving of the head from the blast wind that follows. Again, this is the blast wind. These features, the blast wave and blast wind, are distinct physical aspects of blast exposure. And this distinction that you can clearly distinguish in the video is going to have direct relevance for what happens in the brain.

CHANGE IN HEAD ACCELERATION IS THE KEY

That head motion, specifically head acceleration—and even more importantly, not just the acceleration, but the change in acceleration, or "jolt"—is very important here. If you think about when you've been on a roller coaster, it's the change of acceleration that is really the exciting piece of it—when you take a turn or when you go up and down. It's when you change your acceleration, that is the "jolt," and that is what we need to pay attention to here. The older, predominant theories of what happens during blast exposure are that either it has no effect on the brain—which still many people believe to be true—or that there is some effect on the thorax that causes a "water hammer" effect that is transmitted to the brain by the large blood vessels, the carotid arteries and its tributaries. The water hammer idea didn't make sense to us, first because you would expect to find watershed hemorrhages in specific regions of the brain—and we don't—and second, because the physics don't work out in terms of the timing. We actually measured intracranial pressure using a sensor in the brain, and we didn't see evidence for the water hammer effect (Fig. 5.5A). Further, to have a water hammer effect, you need the vasculature of

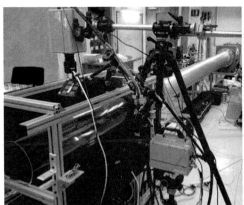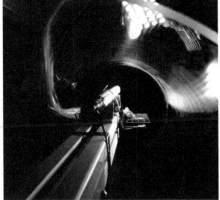

FIG. 5.4 Boston University blast neurotrauma mouse model. No anesthesia or apnea used. There is 100% survival of the mice. (Figure courtesy of Dr. Goldstein.)

the thorax to be intact. We found when we isolate the head—thereby mechanically disrupting the connection between the thorax (and vasculature) and brain—we observed the same blast-induced pressure signals in the brain (Fig. 5.5B). This experiment shows that the water hammer effect—pressure on the thorax that is transmitted to the brain by the large blood vessels—cannot be the mechanism by which a blast pressure wave induces TBI and triggers CTE.

So we concluded the mechanism must be due to something else. Indeed, the mechanism is what I just showed you: motion of the head. One of my graduate students, Mark Wojnarowicz, dubbed the mechanism that we uncovered "the bobblehead effect." The visual associated with head movement of a bobblehead doll conveys the general idea of the type of motion involved, albeit with much greater intensity and faster kinetics in the context of blast exposure. Fig. 5.6 shows the head

moving in time resulting from a single experimental blast exposure in a mouse.

Blast Exposure Triggers Microscopic CTE Pathology but Not Macroscopic Injury

One striking finding about this blast model was that even using the best small animal MRI machines in the country at the Massachusetts Institute of Technology we saw really nothing unusual in the brain. The brains looked normal. Dr. Martha Shenton (Chapter 11) will provide evidence from the literature and from her own lab about what MRI visible changes happen in the brain after various injuries, but if you just look at a standard structural MRI immediately after an injury of the type we have been discussing, I think the overwhelming data are that you don't see much of anything. You have to either use special MRI sequences or other types of techniques to look at a patient with acute, mild TBI and see these

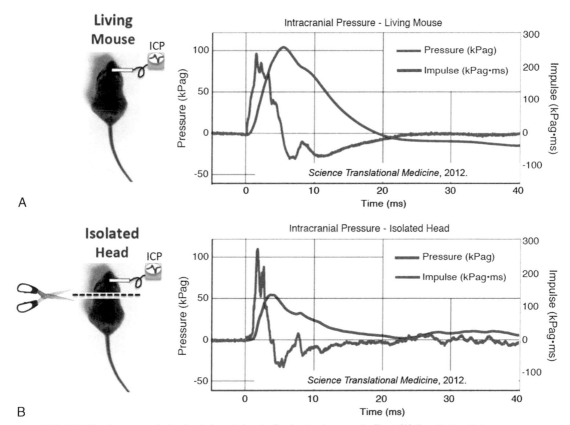

FIG. 5.5 Blast pressure in the brain is not due to the "water hammer" effect. **(A)** Results in a living mouse. **(B)** Results from an isolated head. Note the similarities. (With permission from Goldstein LE, et al. Chronic traumatic encephalopathy in blast-exposed military veterans and a blast neurotrauma mouse model. *Science Translational Medicine*. May 16, 2012;4(134):134ra60.)

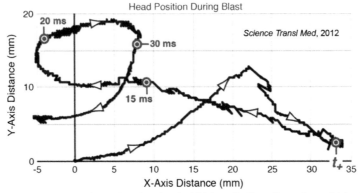

FIG. 5.6 Head position during a blast showing the "bobblehead" effect. Note the multiple changes of acceleration. (With permission from Goldstein LE, et al. Chronic traumatic encephalopathy in blast-exposed military veterans and a blast neurotrauma mouse model. *Science Translational Medicine*. May 16, 2012;4(134):134ra60.)

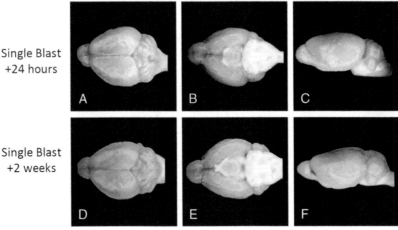

FIG. 5.7 Ex vivo gross pathology after exposure to a single blast. Note there are no signs of contusion, necrosis, hematoma, hemorrhage, or focal injury. (With permission from Goldstein LE, et al. Chronic traumatic encephalopathy in blast-exposed military veterans and a blast neurotrauma mouse model. *Science Translational Medicine*. May 16, 2012;4(134):134ra60.)

injuries. We see the same thing (that is, nothing unusual) in blast-exposed animals. Even when we examined the brains postmortem, they looked entirely normal on the surface (Fig. 5.7). We didn't see contusions, hematomas, or hemorrhage, and we saw no evidence of focal injury immediately after the blast or after 1 day or 2 weeks. The brains looked normal. This result is similar to the data in humans from both the VA and the Department of Defense—we don't see anything by routine structural imaging and we don't see anything grossly in pathology.

However, if you look at the microscopic pathology after a single blast exposure in this mouse model, we see evidence of just about everything that we have seen in the human brains, including evidence of CTE. Our results are in wild-type, nontransgenic mouse, nothing special about these mice. From an evolutionary perspective, mouse brain is similar to the human brain after having only 7 million years to diverge from our common ancestor. In evolutionary time, this is a blink of the eye. In fact, we share most of our genes with the mouse. There is a lot to say about the fact that we see the same pathology in the mouse after a single exposure—including the tauopathy, which we actually thought was not going to happen (Fig. 5.8). We see the tauopathy by the brown staining, as well as by chemistry and other techniques. We have now done a large

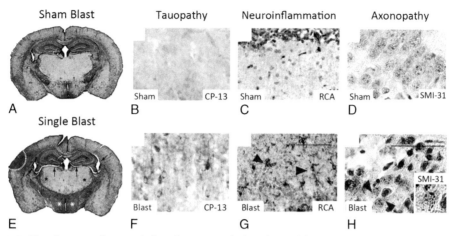

FIG. 5.8 Chronic traumatic encephalopathy neuropathology from a blast neurotrauma mouse model, 2 weeks after a single blast. Note the increased brown staining indicating damage in panels E through H. (With permission from Goldstein LE, et al. Chronic traumatic encephalopathy in blast-exposed military veterans and a blast neurotrauma mouse model. *Science Translational Medicine*. May 16, 2012;4(134):134ra60.)

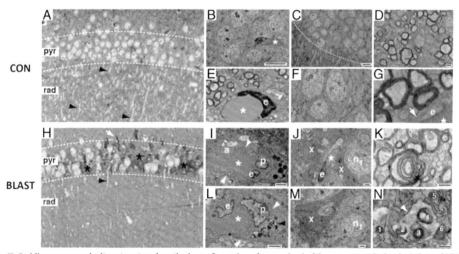

FIG. 5.9 Hippocampal ultrastructural pathology 2 weeks after a single blast traumatic brain injury. (With permission from Goldstein LE, et al. Chronic traumatic encephalopathy in blast-exposed military veterans and a blast neurotrauma mouse model. *Science Translational Medicine*. May 16, 2012;4(134):134ra60.)

analysis with many mice and we see the same findings as in this one example.

Here is one of the reasons why I think we have had such difficulty seeing this injury by standard imaging techniques. This disease starts below the level of light microscopy. The injury starts at the level of ultrastructure, at the level that requires an electron microscope to see, so it's no surprise that it's tough to observe this damage using MRI, which measures, at best, fractions of millimeters (Fig. 5.9).

Fig. 5.10 shows a mouse capillary, the smallest blood vessel in the brain, and a perivascular astrocyte 2 weeks after blast exposure. This is one sick neurovascular unit. There are many things really wrong with it. You can see the capillary just barely hanging on from a structural perspective. There has been a lot of focus on axons and a lot less focus on the microvasculature, but as Dr. McKee and I have shown you, the microvasculature is where the action starts—and indeed persists and appears to progress. You'll hear more about the

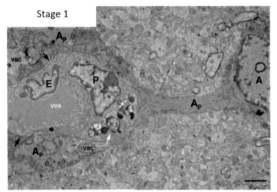

Stage 1

FIG. 5.10 Traumatic brain injury/chronic traumatic encephalopathy-linked ultrastructural microvasculopathy. Image shows electron microscopy 2 weeks after a single blast exposure. *A*, astrocyte; *A$_P$*, astrocytic process; *E*, endothelial cell; *P*, perivascular pericyte; *vac*, vacuole; *ves*, vessel; *arrow* shows lipofuscin granules; bar = 2 μm. (With permission from Goldstein LE, et al. Chronic traumatic encephalopathy in blast-exposed military veterans and a blast neurotrauma mouse model. *Science Translational Medicine*. May 16, 2012;4(134):134ra60.)

importance of the microvasculature from Dr. Diaz-Arrastia (Chapter 12).

Changes in Brain Physiology

So who cares if all that is happening in your brain if it still works well? Well, the answer is that the brain is not working well. Fig. 5.11 shows evidence looking at axonal conduction, which is how messages are carried from one place to another in the brain. Below that is long-term potentiation, which is the fundamental neurobiological substrate of learning and memory. Fig. 5.12 shows mouse learning in action. As you can see, all of these are profoundly affected by this injury—and recall that these effects persist (and appear to progress) following exposure to a single blast.

Speaking of which, I would like to comment on exactly what it means to have "one exposure to a blast." One exposure to a blast does not produce a single injury. Because the head is being moved rapidly back and forth, there are likely multiple injuries related to changes in acceleration because the head is going back and forth, as we discussed before. There is also the "local-focal" issue that depends on how shearing forces associated with this traumatic

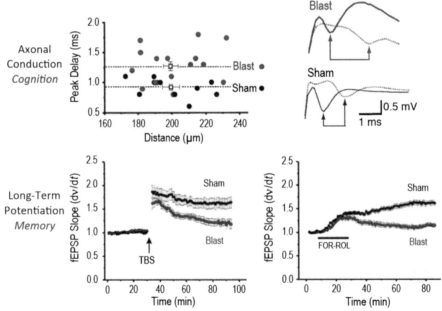

FIG. 5.11 Defective hippocampal axonal conduction and synaptic plasticity affecting speed of cognition and memory function after blast injury. *fEPSP*, field excitatory postsynaptic potential; *FOR-ROL*, forskolin + rolipram; *TBS*, theta-burst stimulation. (With permission from Goldstein LE, et al. Chronic traumatic encephalopathy in blast-exposed military veterans and a blast neurotrauma mouse model. *Science Translational Medicine*. May 16, 2012;4(134):134ra60.)

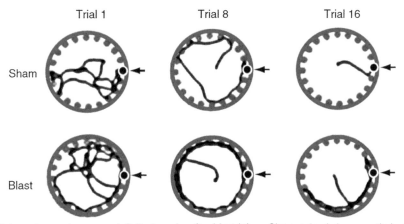

FIG. 5.12 Learning and memory deficits 2 weeks after blast injury. Sham animals improve their ability to find the target in the Barnes maze more quickly than blast-exposed animals. (With permission from Goldstein LE, et al. Chronic traumatic encephalopathy in blast-exposed military veterans and a blast neurotrauma mouse model. *Science Translational Medicine*. May 16, 2012;4(134):134ra60.)

motion interact with the tissue structures and interfaces at any given locus in the brain. So brain injury induced by blast exposure collectively represents many injuries distributed across time (about 10 to 15 ms) and in space. These injuries trigger secondary mechanisms that lead to other brain pathologies, including CTE.

So we are seeing these types of injury that affect memory and cognition after one blast exposure. Note that if we hold the head still and let the blast wave go by and without moving the head, then we don't see these types of injuries and we don't see effects on learning and memory behavior (Fig. 5.13). The bottom line is that it's the head motion that is causing these types of effects.

Relating the Mouse Model to Human Disease

So we know that blast exposure causes rapid movement of the head and this motion—or strictly speaking, the shear forces associated with this motion—is what damages the brain and triggers CTE pathology. Importantly, we are able to see pretty much everything in the mouse model that we see in human cases. We see microvasculopathy, neuroinflammation, myelinated axonopathy, tau proteinopathy, neurodegeneration, behavior deficits, TBI gene expression, and we see changes in the retina of the eye as well. The mouse model is actually very, very, very close to what we observe in humans. So what is happening here is related to the acceleration or change in head acceleration, energy transfer causing focal shear stress, which causes acute tissue

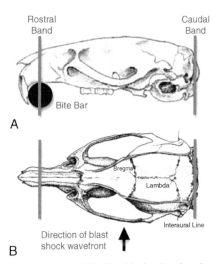

FIG. 5.13 Head immobilization blocks the chronic effects of blast traumatic brain injury (TBI) by blocking the "bobblehead effect." **(A)** Two miniature nylon cable ties were placed to immobilize the head. **(B)** Head fixation blocks the detrimental chronic effects to memory of blast TBI. (With permission from Goldstein LE, et al. Chronic traumatic encephalopathy in blast-exposed military veterans and a blast neurotrauma mouse model. *Science Translational Medicine*. May 16, 2012;4(134):134ra60.)

damage. The question is, how do those things relate? Dr. Rowson was talking about concussion in relation to this disease (Chapter 4). How does concussion relate? Fig. 5.14 shows one model that we developed to try to answer those questions.

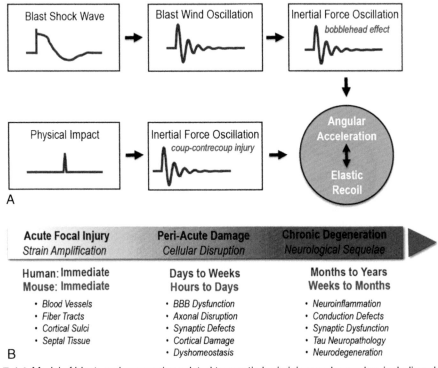

FIG. 5.14 Model of blast- and concussion-related traumatic brain injury and sequelae, including chronic traumatic encephalopathy. (With permission from Goldstein LE, et al. Chronic traumatic encephalopathy in blast-exposed military veterans and a blast neurotrauma mouse model. *Science Translational Medicine.* May 16, 2012;4(134):134ra60.)

CONCLUSIONS: PUTTING IT ALL TOGETHER

Let me spend a minute explaining some of these concepts I've been talking about using a common sense approach. So if I want to punch a hole in the stage, I am better off doing it with a high-heel shoe instead of my flat shoe because of point loading in the former versus distributed loading in the latter. The same thing can happen in the brain whether we use the analogy of that of a golf ball moving due to an impact or a sailboard moving due to a blast of wind. These analogies are relevant to what happens in the head during impact compared to blast. We have recently shown that energy going into the head loads differently in these two cases, even when the resulting head motion is the same. While the gross motion of the head may be the same, these two energy-loading conditions are very different—and set up very different stress fields in the brain. In ongoing work in my laboratory, we have evidence that these differences in injury physics differentiate concussion from brain injury.

In the case of the brain under these mechanical conditions and time regimes, stress concentration will occur in the depths of cortical sulci ("notches"), in and around small blood vessels (filled "holes"), and at interfaces of the gray and white matter in the brain. This is exactly where we see brain pathology associated with acute injury and long-term sequelae, including CTE. The stress concentrations are happening right at these interfaces. If you think about it, this makes sense, because if you have a stress concentration at the base of the sulcus, then it's just a matter of physics that this will be the region of greatest focal trauma. If you put two sulci together you will get a circle, and that is where you get stress concentrations around small blood vessels. Let's be clear—in the time domains of these injuries, the brain does not respond as if it were a gelatinous mass like Jell-O. Rather, the brain is more like a solid material, pliable plastic if you will, and as physics demands of any such material subject to such mechanical forces, stress concentration will occur exactly where we observe the greatest pathology. The laws of physics are exactly that, the law of matter, and as such, apply both inside and outside the skull. It's the law.

We can see this type of force in other aspects of life as well. As you walk down the street you may see a crack in the sidewalk. Cracks in concrete are invariably associated with a notch, hole, interface, or some other structural inhomogeneity that serves as a stress concentrator. You can see the results of the same physics in a cracked hoof of a horse. For the same reason, I have a fracture in a tooth that started as a chip. You can see the same effect on a grander scale in geological fractures. My dad is a civil engineer who specialized in concrete and road building. He used to take me for walks, and if we passed a manhole cover with cracks in the adjacent concrete, he'd point out that the cracks are due to freeze-thaw (or heat) cycles causing stress concentration around the manhole. This is why most manholes nowadays have pliable rings and asphalt around them to dissipate the effects of thermally induced stress concentration. I never thought I would use any of this knowledge, and certainly never thought concrete could be related to the brain—but it is the same thing. (I thanked my dad, by the way.) Fig. 5.15 shows my favorite candy bar, Thin Mints, and if you notice the top of the packaging, you'll see the saw-tooth crenellation in the wrapping—same thing applies to a bag of chips. When you apply opposing force across the notches of the crenellated wrapper, the mechanical force is concentrated at the base. I hope you remember this point: the reason you can open the package is because those little notches concentrate the stress with opposing forces right at the base of the crenulations, and that's how you get into that candy bar or bag of chips—and whatever health consequences follow. It's the same principles at work when the brain gets damaged.

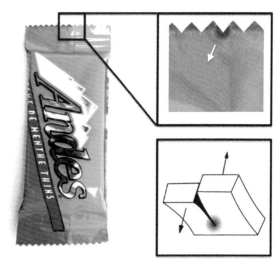

FIG. 5.15 Crenulated edge of candy packaging designed to produce pressure concentrations to aid opening. (Figure courtesy of Dr. Goldstein.)

DISCLOSURES

Dr. Goldstein receives support from NIH (NIA, NINDS), VA, DoD, CDMRP, CENC (DoD-VA), WWE, Crown Family Foundation, Concussion Legacy Foundation, Thermo Scientific, and Boston University.

REFERENCE

1. Goldstein LE, Fisher AM, Tagge CA, et al. Chronic traumatic encephalopathy in blast-exposed military veterans and a blast neurotrauma mouse model. *Science Translational Medicine*. May 16, 2012;4(134):134ra60. http://dx.doi.org/10.1126/scitranslmed.3003716.

CHAPTER 6

Family Panel Discussion

ROBERT A. STERN

Note: Although introduced by name at the conference, in this chapter several family members are anonymous and certain details have been changed or omitted to protect their privacy.

Dr. Stern: It is hard to even describe what it's like being surrounded by these folks, these people whom we refer to as "legacy family donors." These are the people whose loved ones have died and their brains have been examined by Dr. McKee and her team. Yesterday there was a group of 80 family members who were here for a 3-day "huddle." We brought these 80 people together who haven't really known each other but whose lives have been affected by chronic traumatic encephalopathy (CTE) and who've gone through this experience of working with Dr. McKee's team when she gives the diagnosis of the loved one with tender care. You get all those people together, and it's the most profoundly wonderful experience. It's not easy—it's hard for everyone—but it's wonderful. It's wonderful in terms of bonding, of not being alone in a very lonely disease, experience, and journey. It's wonderful because of the sharing of stories, pain, fears, and also laughter. And so it's a very unique type of club. And to be able to be a part of it, in the middle of it, dealing with the science of it, thinking about where we can go next scientifically, and then to be surrounded by these wonderful people is an honor and blessing.

Knowing that this group of people was going to be in town at the same time as this conference, we decided to have a family panel so you can learn from their experiences, so you can take what you've been learning about CTE from this conference and make it personal. We asked these four individuals, and they agreed in order to give a somewhat diverse perspective. Not everyone with CTE played in the National Football League (NFL), and we also have a mixture of spouses and adult children. We wanted you to hear the different types of symptoms that these individuals with CTE had, and to hear the stories from the families who have lived with these individuals. So for the next 45 minutes or so I am going to have each of the family members give a brief outline of their journey, and then I will follow up with questions that I've been aching to ask them all,

and then we can open it up to your questions. These are brave, beautiful souls that I've gotten to know, and I think you will appreciate hearing their stories.

Elizabeth Allardice: First of all, thank you all, all of you who are here from the medical community. I appreciate your interest in learning about the disease CTE that has affected my life in a very personal way, and I hope that you continue to follow the research and help our team here at Boston University (BU) with their research and discovery of solutions for this disease.

My husband was Robert Allardice. His nickname was "Dice" and he played college football at the United States Military Academy at West Point. He started playing football when he was age 12, and in high school he played varsity football, along with varsity wrestling and track and field. He played college football at West Point, where he was a defensive tackle in his junior year. He also did boxing—required in the military academy. In his junior year, he suffered three concussions in 1 week in October, and the following week he had a neck break that resulted in surgery, a fusion of his neck that ended his career as an athlete. He graduated from West Point and was on his way to his first tour of duty in Vietnam, and, while in Germany, he was rear-ended in a traffic accident. He was taken by ambulance and evaluated, and at that point in time his military career was ended honorably. He was given a disability for excessive traumatic brain injury for his West Point time and the traffic accident. In 1970, his medical forms when he was discharged said that he was cognitively intact, but we were worried about the future cognitively.

My husband then went on in life. He was in the sales arena in corporate America and worked in an industry for 30 years in sales and development for a company, retiring in 2006. We had begun to see symptoms of something not being right before that. And these were cognitive things, like inability to process information. At this point he was retired, and I was working full time, and he would go to the grocery store and bring back things we never used. It was difficult trying to figure out why he couldn't make a list. There were other subtle things like that.

We had a number of psychological workups. The first one didn't give us a definitive explanation. The workup that had been done was the neurological workup. There was a period of time, about a year and half, before the next workup. At that workup we found he had executive function difficulties. We knew this already as a family, that he was just not able to process stuff. We had a really tough time. He was a "faller," and I can't even begin to tell you how many times he fell and the trauma associated with those falls.

We had a difficult time in the medical community because nobody could figure out what was going on with him. I think the worst thing for me as an individual was trying to get the medical community to understand that he couldn't process information. If there was a question about pain the answer could be "yes," but "do you want medicine?" That was a separate question, and the two were not connected in his mind. You could ask him, "do you want pancakes for breakfast?" and he would say, "yes," but if you asked him, "what do you want for breakfast?" he had no clue. There was real difficulty processing, even the less complicated things.

From a medical standpoint there was no diagnosis to begin with. When people came to try and help him during his short hospital stays and then during his almost 2 years' stay in the Veterans Affairs (VA) community living center, there wasn't ever the realization, in my opinion, that the caregivers/doctors/staff understood he could not process information in a normal functioning way. For example, when you take someone to the lavatory and you leave them there and think they can push the button to tell someone they want to go back to bed, those who can't process the information will stand there for hours.

I invite you as the medical community, when you're treating someone with brain injury from the past, to pull information from the databank about what is going on with executive functioning and what goes on in the frontal lobes. If there is anything you can do to help—maybe you do not have the answer but at least try to improve the quality of life for your patient. That would be something I could hope for.

My husband died 2 years ago in 2014, and when he died, the first diagnosis from the BU team was CTE stage 3, and the second diagnosis was progressive supranuclear palsy. When he died, he had been stripped of all his dignity. He could do nothing. He couldn't function on his own. He could do absolutely nothing, so it was a very tragic disease for my husband, for me, and for my family as we watched it. We need answers and help. The medical community, together, can help our patients and families with consideration of what quality of life means. Thank you.

First child: I will start at the end and then go back to the beginning very quickly.

My father was in his 70s when he died from a medical disease. Maybe 6 weeks before he died, we were in the hospital and the geriatric internist came in. He was going over my father's charts and he says, "and of course he has dementia," and I said, "he doesn't have dementia," and he said, "I am a geriatric doctor and this my specialty, your father has dementia," and I said, "well, if he has dementia then has always had dementia because he has always been this way."

So that was a few years ago. He was a very early case at BU, when they were working hard to identify brains. We received a "cold call"—I guess his death was announced on the wire—and they called the next day. He never had a diagnosed concussion, and so we assumed he was a control for the study.

He played football when he was in seventh grade in 6-man football and they played both sides—offense and defense—until he was a senior, and then they went into 11-man football. He played 4 years in college. He was also a gifted baseball player, and when he graduated, he was offered professional contracts for both baseball and football. He tried baseball for a summer and decided football would be easier on his relationship with my mom. He had an NFL career as a running back. He played in a number of world championships. He was really proud of his affiliations with some of the greatest athletes of the 20th century.

He was also an amazing carpenter. I remember being a child and doing carpentry with him. He had daughters, no sons, and we played softball and we did carpentry with him. He was patient, methodical, exact, and meticulous. What I now understand was his executive functioning was impeccable. So we learned carpentry from him.

When he was older, sometimes he would go out on Saturday and not come home until Sunday. At the time I thought he was being a big jerk. Now that I hear stories about CTE, I think he simply got into his car and he forgot what he was going to do and just went on his merry way to someplace he remembered. It was a small city and the cops knew him, I am sure, and everyone always managed it. We heard rumors that he couldn't find work eventually because he was rumored to be an alcoholic. I don't have a problem with the idea that he was an alcoholic, but I didn't see him drink. So now I think it may have been all CTE. He left his last job, and he kind of wandered around. My mother ultimately left him.

I remember his losing his temper so violently and so off the wall that he was terrifying. This kind of trauma is happening to children and mothers. It is real. So when you have someone coming into your office and the woman seems crazy, she is feeling crazy because she is traumatized and she is trying to hold together this speeding train with its wheels falling off as it's moving.

I finally just want to say I am someone who didn't want to believe the diagnosis was true. My dad was raised in a small town, and he played football to bring the whole family out of poverty and to be on a path to middle class wholesomeness. I wanted Dr. Stern to be crazy and my dad to be an anomaly. I didn't want this diagnosis to be real—but it is real. Please be careful when people like this come in, they are a special breed. They hide stuff, they are stoic, and they are extraordinary—so don't let them fool you!

Mary Hawkins: That's my husband, Rip Hawkins. He started playing football in military high school, and he played as an offensive lineman as well as a defensive middle linebacker. He would never tell football stories until someone would pull them out of him. He was such a humble man. But one of the stories he would tell when people would ask was the incident when he was hit so hard that his helmet cracked in half. He provides the most vivid account of that concussion. He described it as the hair on the back of his neck standing up.

He went to college where he played as an offensive lineman (center) as well as a defensive middle linebacker. He was drafted in the second round for an NFL team in the 1960s and played for 5 years. During the off-season he attended law school. At the end of 5 years they said, "do you want to be a lawyer or football player?" He had to choose, and he chose law. For him, defending justice was what his life was about. He loved football and was passionate about it, but he made that choice. His wife at the time was suffering with mental illness and made multiple suicide attempts. Over the next 5 years, he was raising two children and going to law school in the process of keeping her alive. At the end of 5 years, she was successful in her attempt to commit suicide.

He died at the age of 76. During his life, he was initially diagnosed with postconcussive dementia; no real specific diagnoses, but just labeled as "dementia." About a year before his death, a neurologist says he exhibited all the signs of Lewy body dementia; however, upon the examination of his brain at BU they found he did not have Lewy body but stage 4 CTE.

I guess what I just want to say about his experience personally and professionally is that high cognitive and social reserve can fool people. He had the smooth southern accent, wit, and personality that could charm your socks off. If you were the fact checker as the wife, you knew the story wasn't right, but he could still wag that finger like the district attorney he was with confidence, even when the facts weren't correct.

A month before his death, there was a seizure and a series of multiple falls. He sustained a subdural hematoma with aphasia and was admitted to the intensive care unit, then a trauma unit. He was discharged to a memory care unit for a 3-day respite stay. At the memory care unit, he sustained a total of five severe falls—one with very obvious injuries. I was never informed of the incidents; they were not documented, nor was a physician notified. We elected to take him home where hospice was started and I cared for him until he died 10 days later. Until then, up until the memorial service, all our friends were stunned that this man had any diagnosis that would resemble dementia. He was a master of disguise. Publicly, he was as charming and articulate as you could imagine—until he wasn't. He could carry it off during a social situation and be the life of the party, and then 5 minutes into the ride home he would have a meltdown because he didn't know where he was.

I think that one of my pleas to you, as medical practitioners, would be for your compassion and understanding for the family members and the care partners. As authentic partners, often we see and are aware of things far before any diagnostic assessment can detect them. Having belief and confidence that you, as the care providers, will support the care partners as well as the patient is essential.

Third spouse: My husband died at the age of 66. He suffered with this disease probably 16 years. I tried to keep him at home the whole time, but obviously I needed help. I received help from some family. I also put him in respite care. He would get kicked out, and then he went to mini-psych wards. It was a horrific journey.

He started playing football at age 10. In high school he played linebacker and defensive end. He played both defense and offense. He went to college and he was on their national championship team. He played defensive tackle, and he was smaller than most of the guys. Back then they didn't make them the way they do now. He was like 5′10″, and he went against these guys that were 300 pounds, and his way of hitting was that he had leverage and shoulder strength so he would get under people and rammed his head into their chest. And they taught you to ram your head into the chest. It was violent as it is now.

He died with stage 4 CTE. He didn't have any other health issues, nothing. He didn't have high blood pressure. He didn't have high cholesterol. He was totally physically healthy except for his brain. He just lost his mind. When he died, his death certificate says death from traumatic brain injury not from pneumonia, nothing else. So he died similarly to people who have Alzheimer's disease (AD).

We were married 37 years, and we have two children. In 1998, he started showing irritability, short temper, forgetfulness, and anger. He would throw things. Let me back up. He taught school. He had a master's degree in fine arts. He taught school at a university for 40 years. He loved to talk, and he was a gifted speaker. Well, when he lost his language and lost his ability to do math, I knew something was wrong. So I went to his school and I said he needs to take a medical leave of absence. I became his voice. He could not process; he would look at me to finish sentences. It was very uncomfortable because people thought I was being the bossy wife. I was just trying to take care of him. He totally lost his executive function.

So the journey for us is in trying to support your loved one. It changes you to lose your husband. You lose your friend. You don't have anybody to talk to. So you're caring for this person that you are totally dedicated to, but you're not getting anything back.

The first neurologist said that he had mild cognitive disorder and probably caused from football. So then he sends me to a second neurologist; she said it's definitely Alzheimer's, and she is an Alzheimer's researcher so that's probably why she said that. And then I kept saying he doesn't have Alzheimer's. It doesn't run in his family, and it doesn't run in his genetics. They didn't believe me, so I got a neurologist that works with football players; he said he probably has CTE but you won't know until he dies and sure enough he had stage 4 CTE.

One of my goals is to make people aware of CTE because nobody is listening. They don't want to hear it, they don't want to believe it, and everyone says it's Alzheimer's. If you can figure out a way to differentiate between the two, you will help the patient and caregiver. Another thing he had was headaches. I don't know if it's true, but I was told in one of my conferences that CTE patients get headaches and AD patients don't. I don't know if that's true or not but my husband had headaches for a long time. Thank you.

Dr. Stern: We just heard so many different versions of the same story. And part of that similarity is because the diagnosis is typical. Whether you (referring to first child) saw a guy who was always this kind of person and then someone is saying to you that he has dementia and

you're maybe not even being aware that there has been some kind of decline or it was hard to tell because he has always been in your adult life something different. You (referring to Elizabeth Allardice) were given no real diagnosis, and he kept falling and nobody picked up on it, and it ended up that he had dual diagnoses of CTE and progressive supranuclear palsy. Then he (referring to Mary Hawkins) was diagnosed with dementia with Lewy bodies because all the signs looked just like that clinically. And then you (referring to the third spouse) had, I think, one of the more common situations. You had to find a diagnosis, and Alzheimer's disease is the most common. You were told it must be Alzheimer's, and it wasn't. The one thing that brings you all together is that you were dealing with something different from what most caregivers go through. Yes, there are caregiver issues that caregivers of AD patients experience, but for that they can read and get support from the AD community and AD support groups. (Turning to the audience) The experience of caring for someone with CTE, which you just heard about, is very different. And one *very small* issue is that these are *very big* guys, and you have issues of them being kicked out of facilities and being aggressive and you are not even able to pick them up when they fall. So you are dealing with some situations that are similar to those of AD caregivers, but you are also dealing with some very different situations.

I would now like to ask, were you surprised when you were on that phone call and you were given the diagnosis of CTE from Dr. McKee?

Elizabeth Allardice: Well, I had an interesting situation with my husband's disease, because the surgeon who operated on my husband at West Point when he was in college remained a friend of the family all through the years. So when he and we started seeing symptoms of something different in my husband, we asked him what he thought. And he was able to be that one doctor in all the doctors we saw who said it was related to his concussions. He was the only doctor in all that time who said it was the concussions.

First child: I was surprised. I didn't want to believe it.

Dr. Stern: He was a control.

First child: He was a control in my mind. He never had a recorded concussion, and I was not interested in CTE. I could guarantee we wanted to preserve our football hero who played with legends. I didn't want him to have CTE.

Mary Hawkins: I guess learning that it was CTE surprised me, even when he did have all the classic symptoms and signs of Lewy body dementia. It is not an easy diagnosis to make. Most people would go under the umbrella diagnosis of dementia in general.

But I suppose at that point it didn't matter to me any-more what the label was. I knew we were dealing with something that was real. But there was comfort in knowing there was a label and a name for it.

First child: I just want it to be psychiatric—if any-thing. I assumed there was probably some type of attachment disorder, or it was some type of trauma response, PTSD maybe. I decided a long time ago what was going on with my dad. I think that there may also be misdirection from the patient, because when they come in to see the doctor they are great about talking about themselves because that's all they can remem-ber. And we are all accustomed to athletes talking about themselves, or people really only wanting them to talk about themselves, and so they seem chatty and gregarious and not truly impaired. Interpersonally impaired—not reciprocal or mutual maybe in the way they interact—but not brain impaired.

Third spouse: I was not surprised. Making the video I had trouble deciding whether to show my husband in his condition. I didn't want to hurt his dignity, but it has been a year and half now and I am really getting angry. I am willing to show it, and you will see more in the future. My niece made the first one, and it was only 5 minutes. The new video is 10 minutes, and it shows how he was hitting me. There are many more incidents and it was alarming. That person was not my husband because my husband was a gentle giant. He majored in art. He was sweet. He was compassionate and lov-ing. You can see in the video in the doctor's waiting room he was hitting me, but at the same time he was also patting me, so he still knew love. I don't know if you can categorize love as an executive function, but he was still sympathetic and compassionate and he never lost those qualities and he knew me until the end. And 2 weeks before he died, he stood at the kitchen sink and wanted to die and then he did. He was tired.

Bob Stern: All of you experienced such difficult moments. What were some of them? What was the most difficult thing you experienced?

Elizabeth Allardice: I think for me it was that when we went to the neurologist initially and did the whole neurological workup were told that there was noth-ing cognitively showing up abnormal. Then there was the period of time between that initial evaluation and the follow-up one when we were told that there was a deficit. The cognitive deficits had grown worse since the initial evaluation. And so during that period of time in between I thought he was simply being a jerk. I thought that for some strange reason he no longer loved me, and that he wanted to end our marriage. He decided he was no longer going to shave or bathe. He

was just being vicious. It was the first time I ever heard him shout. Even with all of these sorts of things I heard nothing from the medical community that there was something wrong going on, so I was left with feeling like something was inadequate in our life and that for me was the worst part of the disease.

First child: I think the worst was the isolation and shame. I remember before the diagnosis the isolation and shame and the fear of asking for help. In the end he became very withdrawn and he was quiet, and he became so withdrawn and I quit returning his calls because he kept calling to ask how school was and I would tell him I am not in school and you never listen. But I think that the worst was the isolation and shame and thinking that he didn't care. And look, my fam-ily was torn apart from this disease. My father met my mother at age 15 and they got married when she was 17, and they were married for 46 years. She had to leave him to save herself. Our family was destroyed. I could go on, but I won't.

Mary Hawkins: I think the toughest things came in the different stages. Initially, I think it was probably learning how to not take it personally—which is dif-ficult to do when this is your partner, your companion, and your soul mate. Then it was the energy it took to continuously sidestep the behavior that is not him—that behavior is not my husband, not the man who loves me. Again isolation. Also the disbelief of loved ones. It was difficult when it became unsafe for me to sleep in the same bed because the rapid eye movement sleep disorder resulted in violent dreams. It was diffi-cult sharing his problems with family members who just didn't want to accept this and so I must have been making it up. Where do you go with that and how do you reconcile it? Those were tough times. I think the ambiguous losses of him being there, but not there—having a husband and no marriage was difficult. For years, I was in that anticipatory state of hypervigilance: How can I attempt to offset the next behavior? How can I plan? How can I anticipate? How do I keep him safe, me safe, and people on the road safe? The energy consumed was absolutely exhausting. I think just now, in a little over a year after his death, I am just now just starting to emerge, to recover normalcy in my sleep pat-terns, recalibrating my life, and having the strength and courage to voice this experience for him and for other care partners. The physical and emotional toll of this disease on the care partners is a component that is woe-fully underserved.

Third spouse: One of the hardest parts of our jour-ney is that we moved eight times in 2½ years looking for a facility, for memory care. As I told you, he was asked to leave about six places. I would put him in respite and then I would take him home. I wanted him to stay home. And it's hard to find a personal caregiver. It's too expensive, and even the facilities were expensive, they are 5000 to 6000 dollars a month. But moving eight times trying to find a place where he can fit, it was really difficult. I don't know if some of you know this; I was so torn apart I didn't know what to do. He had been to the psych ward. He was on these drugs and antipsychotics that made him hallucinate. He hit the mini blinds and the walls, and he would try to tear the blinds. He would yell at people outside. He was losing his mind. Well, I got him a marijuana joint—we were from the 60s and I know he used to smoke marijuana—he took two puffs and sat in the chair and looked at the TV, and I said, "Oh my, I found the answer." The next week I was driving to Colorado in my truck and he was hitting my truck and he would try to open the door at 70 mph. So we got to Colorado and I got him a medical marijuana license. We are in the motel and he locks himself into the motel room when I took my dog to the bathroom and he couldn't open the door, so, long story short, he went to a facility and a week later they kicked him out. I was in another state picking up my stuff, and they call me saying he was in the ER, come and get him. They took him like a criminal: put him on a gurney, strapped him in, and here is my husband. He had a master's in art and he was a sweet man. I finally got there; he had one sock on, they couldn't get him to eat, and they had five policemen holding him down and they shot him with a drug. So I decided to leave and I said "he is off all his drugs." So I go back to the hotel to get him off all his drugs, and I got the right medical marijuana oil and for 7 months gave that to him twice a day and he had at least some sort of quality of life. I knew he was dying, so why not let him be stoned, who cares? He was smiling and then he died. So if you have any patients that need medical marijuana, you should think about it. And the medical community, the care communities, and the memory care communities, they are all broken.

Mary Hawkins: I want to add one more thing. The frustration I experienced in getting an accurate assessment and diagnosis so we could begin treatment and care was compounded for me. I have been in the field of medicine in many different areas for 40 years, and I couldn't imagine what it must have been like for these families who didn't have a medical background to help them navigate and get information. I think having a junkyard dog mentality—demanding and asking for things—the physicians resented me for it. They also resented me for sharing with them my knowledge,

especially those when we lived in a rural area. They didn't like that Dr. Google was my first opinion. So often the interactions between my husband and the doctors was more of the physician wanting to know more about his glory days of football, not what his symptoms were at that time. And since his self-report was not reliable, I would have to call the doctor later and have the real talk. That was one of the aspects of communication I didn't share with my husband. The communication in our marriage was always based on honesty and integrity, but I found myself in the position of being a creative storyteller and telling "fiblets" that were required in order to protect him, myself, and others.

Even though there were horror stories, we were graced. The last year and half of his life we went to this small town in Wyoming, moving from a ranch because it became unsafe. He would tip over tractors, leave the gates open letting the horses out, water flooding the stalls, nearly burned down the house a couple of times... I could go on and on. We moved to a small town and found an angel of a geriatrician who traveled 60 miles on a Sunday morning with her husband and 4-year-old child to go to the memory care unit to do an assessment after my husband fell five times. We made a decision to pull him physically out of the facility (they couldn't find a wheelchair) and bring him home for hospice. She then followed with three home visits and came to his memorial service. That's the kind of caring we were so hungry for and I am so grateful that we have a memory of the best.

Bob Stern: I have a hard question for you. Football was a really big part of each of your husbands', or your father's, life. Knowing what you know now, if he knew of his diagnosis, looking back, do you think he would say, "I would do it again"?

Elizabeth Allardice: For my husband, I think from the moment he went to West Point it was all about duty, honor, and country. He loved the game that allowed him to go there. He loved his colleagues. Those folks were with him to the very end, and he wouldn't make a different decision.

First child: He would have played baseball.

Mary Hawkins: I think he would have still played football.

Third spouse: I think he wouldn't have played football. He loved art more than he did football. I would like to say he wouldn't have played football from the orthopedic issues; he had serious pain issues and he told my nephew not to play football.

Dr. Stern: Take that to the next step. He told your nephew to not play. How about each of you? Dr. McKee and I are asked on a daily basis, "would you let your son play football?" We try to get out of answering that. If you had a son or a grandson interested in football, what would you do?

Elizabeth Allardice: I think it's really difficult to think through because of the benefits of sports for our children. I would be very proactive holding off on any participation in sports until later age. I think there should be no Pop Warner football and no sports.

Dr. Stern: No sports or no hitting of the head?

Elizabeth Allardice: No sports, period, until the child was at least in high school.

First child: Over my dead body is the answer, and part two is, of course, they would do sports. I was an athlete, I played basketball, I was a soccer coach, and I am a runner.

Dr. Stern: How about football?

First child: Over my dead body!

Mary Hawkins: Personal choice is such a hot topic. There are risks and benefits. I know there are benefits of the camaraderie of sports, the teamwork, and so the question is, "how can we minimize the risk?" I grew up with football with five brothers. I was told if I wanted to play I couldn't cry. So can we do it safely? I don't know. I wouldn't encourage grandchildren to play, certainly not at a young age.

Third spouse: Absolutely not! There are so many other sports. I played soccer for 20 years competitively. I am getting ready to donate my brain. I didn't start playing until age 25 so hopefully my brain was developed by 25 and, who knows, I may not have damage. Football is so violent to me. Football is also athletic—you can watch it and feel like you're a part of it. But the violence is bad. I can't watch it anymore. My answer is no. No to football!

Bob Stern: So do people in the audience have any burning questions?

Question from Audience: First of all, I want to thank you all. I want to thank the leaders, but I especially want to thank you for adding a personal dimension. One of the things I am certainly hearing from you is that you would advise us to listen better as practitioners. I am certainly hearing the frustrations with the diagnosis. Even before we had biomarkers for Alzheimer's disease we had support groups. We had various ways that people could seek support. Now CTE is not as recognized as AD. I am interested in your perspective of what you found most helpful in terms of support systems, and where we as practitioners could most help patients that we see who might have CTE and their families. I am interested in what organizations exist for

CTE. Or is BU the only place for us to send the people we see with possible CTE?

Mary Hawkins: I am currently beginning the process of developing a website for CTE care partners. Where I have personally found support has been in the last 2 days during our legacy family donor "huddle." We don't have to do anything other than to just tell our stories and everyone understands. The first step is knowledge, and if knowledge is power, then in understanding and in community there is hope. This is a situation in which we know that there is just one trajectory. And that is why I would like to develop a website. We would then form local "huddles" and support learning the skills for communication and for care. And I know others are working on other types of groups. So it's in the works.

Another answer from the panel: I would say we need a support group. I started going to a 12-step group for families of alcoholics because I found their behaviors—the unpredictably of their behaviors—more similar to my experience than those of Alzheimer's disease. The tools you learn are helpful—so much living with the disease is gaining the tools and managing your own feelings of what they are doing. A big piece is managing them, but our own self-care is also important. I mean, our self-care goes out the window with this disorder. Spouses of those with this disease are getting no sleep. There is a lot of that. There is a group that's launching publicly called After the Impact Fund. It is for treating military veterans and NFL players with cognitive impairment and brain injury and there is a peer-to-peer aspect to it. They want to be a sort of virtual case manager, I guess, since there is so little out there yet in terms of guidance. So essentially, they are looking to have a piece of paper to be developed so the family can assess what is also going on. Baseline questions like: Do you eat regularly? Do you sleep 8 hours? What are your obstacles to eating regularly and getting high-quality sleep? All the kinds of things that complicate diagnosing and treating brain injury. Same questions for the care partners! Sometimes they seem more unglued than the guy. We are also looking for tests that would show you a picture of cognitive impairment that might be associated with football. So we are looking for a scaffold to help you, the doctors, so that you can help us. We are hoping to create a 3-day assessment that is funded. We are trying to create a clearinghouse of doctors that believe this disease exists. Like Dr. McKee mentioned earlier, the first step is acknowledging CTE exists. It does exist. So we need to have these lists for each region of the country: if you live in region X go see this guy or woman.

Dr. Stern: Concussion Legacy Foundation is an amazing organization, and right now it is trying to bring together all the different potential resources out there to become a clearinghouse for people to find information and perhaps, moving forward, bring together individuals who would create the support groups. So it's just beginning, and I think it's happening because of the strength of folks like you who are doing it on your own. You have taught us that support groups are critical. It starts like you said: AD support groups have been around for a while, but with this disease it is very different. There are different care partners, there are different types of symptoms—including physical symptoms—and the backgrounds of these guys are also different.

Comment from Audience: I just wanted to say thanks for all you are doing. I appreciate your helping Dr. Stern and Dr. McKee in educating us. I think you hit roadblocks because you were driving ahead of the medical community. I know from personal experience that it's hard to believe in things, that they exist, until it is shown that they do. So when I found my first blast injury cases I didn't believe that they were having trouble. And then I thought, "maybe I should believe in something I didn't think was real." I agree with everything you are trying to do to educate people, and I think this combined approach in this conference of scientists, clinicians, and care partners is helpful.

Dr. Stern: Thank you so very much for sharing your stories!

CHAPTER 7

Genetics of Chronic Traumatic Encephalopathy

JESSE MEZ • BOBAK ABDOLMOHAMMADI

INTRODUCTION

Thank you, Dr. Andrew Budson, for organizing this conference, and thank you, Drs. Bob Stern, Ann McKee, and Bob Cantu, for leading the event. I'm not quite the rock star that Drs. McKee, Stern, and Cantu are, so I only get 20 minutes to speak with you, but honestly, when we were planning this course I couldn't imagine speaking for a full hour because we know so little about the genetics of chronic traumatic encephalopathy (CTE). That being said, we have a lot of exciting plans for genetic analyses in the future. I hope that we will continue having this course and that in the future when I give this talk, it will focus less on what we have planned and more on what we have learned. In any case, here is the outline of the lecture. First, we will discuss the motivation for conducting genetic studies of CTE and the methodologies for these studies. We will spend some time talking about previous findings, and then I will discuss future directions for genetic studies. Lastly, we will discuss the ethics of genetic testing.

WHY GENETICS MAY BE IMPORTANT FOR CTE

As Dr. Stern and Dr. Lee Goldstein said yesterday, I am a clinician first and foremost. Beyond genetics, I am also involved in the clinical evaluation of our brain donors via interviews with their families. Here are two cases from the Understanding Neurologic Injury and Traumatic Encephalopathy (UNITE) study that demonstrate why genetics is important in CTE. We have a 28-year-old whose initials are PC and a 25-year-old whose initials are MK. Both played very similar amounts of football—17 years for PC and 16 years for MK. PC started a little bit later and he ended up playing semi-pro football, while MK started earlier and played through college. MK is actually a case we published in *JAMA Neurology* recently.[1] They both played the same positions—linebacker and special teams. PC had minimal, if any, symptoms, maybe very mild behavioral

or mood symptoms in his mid-20s but on the whole looked like most 20-something-year-olds. MK, on the other hand, starting in college, had pretty substantial mood, behavioral, and cognitive symptoms that didn't allow him to finish his college education. MK also stopped playing football in college because the symptoms were so severe (Fig. 7.1).

Neuropathologically, only MK had CTE (Fig. 7.1). PC's brain wasn't entirely normal, but did not have evidence of CTE. The pathologists found mild ventricular enlargement, perivascular heme-laden macrophages in the frontal white matter, isolated neurofibrillary tangles (NFTs) in the nucleus basalis of Meynert, and rare phosphorylated-tau (ptau) neurites in the locus coeruleus. There was a little bit of tau, but it wasn't enough for a CTE diagnosis. On the other hand, MK had very flagrant CTE for a 25-year-old. He had stage 3 CTE. There was mild ventricular enlargement and hippocampal atrophy and ptau NFTs, neurites, and astrocytes around small blood vessels at the sulcal depths of the frontal and temporal lobes. So we have two guys who had similar exposure and age at death, but had very different CTE neuropathology. It suggests that there are other risk factors at play, as well as age and exposure—very possibly genetic risk factors.

Why should we study genetic risk in CTE? Genes that increase the risk of CTE may help us understand the etiology and biological mechanisms behind the disease. Genetic studies may also aid in counseling contact sport athletes of their risk of developing CTE and may provide targets for disease-modifying drugs for CTE. Therapies that target genes identified through genome-wide association studies (GWAS) ultimately are twice as likely to go to market as those that aren't identified through GWAS, so it's an important potential avenue for drug targets.

METHODOLOGIES

I am going to spend a while talking about methodologies—partly because we are still generating data and

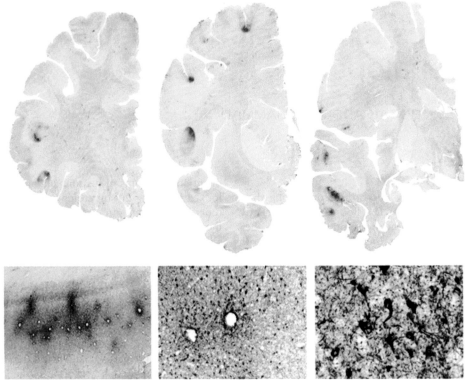

FIG. 7.1 MK, a 25-year-old college football player, died with symptomatic stage II chronic traumatic encephalopathy (CTE). Evidence of stage II CTE. Note that it is easy to see the brown-staining tau in the depths of the sulci on the top images. Bottom images, left to right, show perivascular phospho-tau deposition at increasingly high magnification. (Images courtesy of Dr. McKee.)

don't have a lot of results, but also because we put a lot of thought into devising the right way to design genetic studies. For diseases with complex inheritance patterns, which CTE most likely does, we typically see small effect sizes and we do a lot of statistical tests across the genome, giving us a big multiple-testing problem. We have to come up with the right study design and create statistical approaches so that we can maximize our power.

Choosing Controls

With that in mind, the first thing I'd like to talk about is choosing controls. This is an important concept that Drs. McKee and Stern talked a bit about. All cases of neuropathologically confirmed CTE had exposure to repetitive head impacts (RHI), suggesting RHI is a necessary condition for CTE pathology to develop.

As a brief aside, this statement here is an incredibly strong statement—that we will see CTE only in cases with exposure to RHI—and it brings to mind other diseases where exposure plays a really big role. For instance, there is a small subset of people who aren't

exposed to cigarette smoking who go on to develop chronic obstructive pulmonary disease, and there is small subset of people who aren't exposed to asbestos who still go on to develop mesothelioma. We have by now looked at 200-plus cases neuropathologically, and we reviewed the literature on the disease and we still have never seen a CTE case that didn't have RHI exposure. Again, this doesn't mean it can't happen, but it is with what we know about the exposure in mind that we designed our genetic studies. Ideal controls for genetic studies of CTE should be exposed to RHI, but should not have CTE pathology. Unfortunately, few of these controls have come to autopsy. Given the aforementioned concepts of small effect sizes and many statistical tests to do genetic analyses, we need a large number of controls. So, we really need an alternate approach.

In Alzheimer's disease, most of our controls in genetic studies are clinically asymptomatic but haven't been neuropathologically examined. We know Alzheimer's disease pathology is probably present for 15 to 20 years before manifesting itself symptomatically, so there is

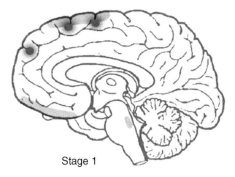

Stage 1

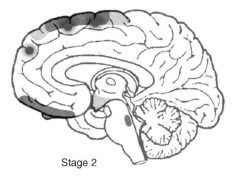

Stage 2

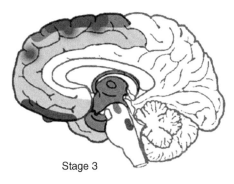

Stage 3

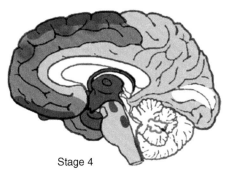

Stage 4

some level of misclassification in AD genetic studies, and we've still been quite successful at identifying new variants. With the AD model in mind, we have alternative possibilities for CTE where we can look at living subjects that we know have been exposed to RHI but who are without clinical symptoms. We can also consider older subjects who are cognitively normal, but we don't know about their RHI exposure. There are a lot of these subjects from our AD genetic studies. Most of them probably haven't played contact sports. Even if they had the genetic background to develop CTE, they would not develop the disease because they were not exposed. In this setting we would have even more misclassification, which would reduce our power and introduce bias. With that being said, increasing our numbers substantially might more than make up for the power loss from the misclassification. While misclassification can introduce bias, it is typically a bias toward the null, so we probably would not identify false positives.

Endophenotypes

Another way of getting more power in genetic studies is to look at endophenotypes rather than just looking at cases and controls. An endophenotype is a measurable intermediate phenotype that is generally closer to the action of the gene than the disease status. Endophenotypes tend to exhibit a higher genetic signal to noise ratio, and while our numbers are small, we are very comprehensive in terms of our phenotypic characterization of our subjects. We don't just measure whether they have CTE or not—we have their pathological stage and semiquantitative NFT counts as well (Fig. 7.2). Our neuropathologists look region by region within the brain and semiquantitatively determine how much pathology is there. Above and beyond that, we have a new slide scanner where we can quantitate how many tangles are there in each anatomic region or throughout the brain.

Clinically, we look at the age of symptom onset, which can give us more power. We can tease out clinical symptoms by looking at behavior/mood vs. cognitive symptoms and also through various imaging techniques. These include MRI, tau PET, and FDG PET, along with cerebrospinal fluid biomarkers.

FIG. 7.2 Neuropathological progression of chronic traumatic encephalopathy by stage. (With permission from Stein TD, Alvarez VE, McKee AC. Chronic traumatic encephalopathy: a spectrum of neuropathological changes following repetitive brain trauma in athletes and military personnel. *Alzheimer's Research & Therapy*. 2014;6(1):4.)

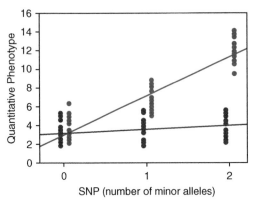

FIG. 7.3 Example of a qualitative gene by environment interaction observed under two environmental conditions (e.g., exposed, red, vs. unexposed, blue). The single-nucleotide polymorphism effect is observed only in the exposed group where the minor allele drives up expression of the phenotype. (Adapted from Idaghdour Y, Awadalla P. Exploiting gene expression variation to capture gene–environment interactions for disease. *Frontiers in Genetics*. 2013;3. http://dx.doi.org/10.3389/fgene.2012.00228.)

Repetitive Head Impacts Exposure Metrics

The next point I want to make concerns our RHI exposure measures. RHI exposure is incredibly important for our genetic studies. Including some sort of measure of exposure is important as a covariate because it explains a lot of the variance in our CTE outcomes. In addition, it is possible that the exposure interacts with genetic risk factors. We may be able to identify genetic factors that may not have main effects but do have interaction effects with exposure. For these reasons, we have made a really concerted effort to understand exposure. We collect a comprehensive exposure history from all our subjects, and we are utilizing helmet sensor data from recent football players and extrapolating that data to our former football players. From these data, we can derive a cumulative measure of exposure that we can use in our genetic model. We recently published the Cumulative Hit Index (CHI),[2] which we can use for genetic studies in living subjects. We also have a paper that is in review right now looking at something pretty similar to the CHI, cumulative lifetime impacts which we can use for genetic studies in our brain donor subjects.

Gene by Environment Interactions

The next point is about gene by environment interactions. When we are talking about gene by environment interaction, we are looking at the joint effect of genes with environmental factors that can't be explained by their separate marginal effects. An example that is easy

to understand is phenylketonuria (PKU). Children with PKU have a genetic mutation that leads to an enzyme deficiency, so that they cannot break down phenylalanine. When affected kids don't eat phenylalanine, they are not exposed and display few clinical symptoms. When they do ingest phenylalanine, they cannot convert phenylalanine to its by-product and they become quite impaired.

In our setting, we are interested in whether an allele has a different effect at different levels of exposure, either qualitatively or quantitatively. Qualitatively, it is an all or nothing phenomenon. If a person isn't exposed to RHI, regardless of their genetic background, they won't develop CTE. If they are exposed, they would develop the disease if they have the genetic background. You can also think about it quantitatively, where we look at different levels of exposure and different levels of phenotypic outcomes, but it is not an all or nothing phenomenon (Fig. 7.3).

This statistical interaction may be related to, but is different from, a biological interaction. In a biological interaction, you have physical contact between two or more factors, usually at the cellular or molecular level. You could have a biological interaction that leads to a statistical interaction, but that is not necessarily always the case.

With gene by environment interactions, you have a lot of challenges. Power and sample size need to be accounted for in the same way as in most genetic studies, possibly even more so. A conservative rule of thumb is that you need four times the number of subjects to identify a gene by environment interaction as you would a main genetic effect. Another issue pertains to including exposure in your model instead of just looking at genetic risk. This makes your model more susceptible to selection bias and confounding. Genetic studies don't usually suffer from these issues given that there isn't really a cause of one's genetic background that could lead to confounding. But once you introduce the exposure, there could be a cause of the exposure, such as where you grow up—football is bigger in some places than others—or your innate ability, which could lead to problems from confounding.

Epigenetics

Another way that the environment can impact your genes is through epigenetics (Fig. 7.4). Epigenetics is defined as a modification to the genome that doesn't alter the primary DNA sequence but leads to changes in gene expression. We know most about DNA methylation, but there are other types of modifications as well, like histone modifications, chromatin remodeling, and microRNAs. Basically, what can happen is

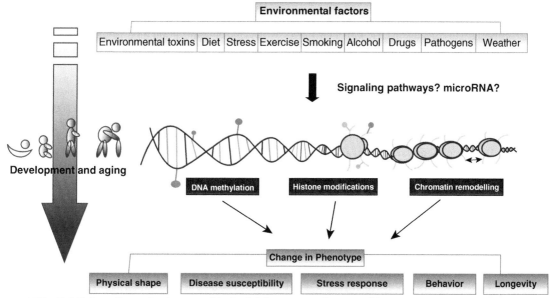

FIG. 7.4 Epigenetic mechanisms provide the link between environmental factors and phenotypical changes. (With permission from Tammen, et al. *Molecular Aspects of Medicine*. 2013.)

that an environmental risk factor can induce these changes in gene expression. We've seen this specifically with DNA methylation. A really interesting example is from McGowan et al.[3] where they found that the hippocampus from postmortem suicide victims who suffered childhood abuse had different DNA methylation of the neuron-specific glucocorticoid receptor (NR3C1) promoter compared with the hippocampus from postmortem suicide victims who did not suffer childhood abuse. These methylations can actually be passed on either mitotically or meiotically, so you can actually pass it on, in theory, from parent to child.

IMPLICATED GENES

APOE

APOE is the genetic risk factor with the largest effect size for sporadic Alzheimer's disease, so those in the neurodegenerative community obviously know that *APOE* is incredibly important. It codes for the primary cholesterol transporter in the brain, and there are three alleles: ε2, ε3, and ε4. They are determined by two single-nucleotide polymorphisms (SNPs). ε4 is the allele that confers an increased risk for Alzheimer's disease. In 1995, Richard Mayeux published a paper in *Neurology* that showed that traumatic brain injury (TBI) was only associated with Alzheimer's disease in the setting of an *APOE* ε4 allele.[4] Lots of people have since tried

to replicate this finding with limited success, but it is nonetheless why we started to get interested in *APOE* as a risk factor in traumatic brain injury.

There is an incredible amount of literature looking at *APOE* and outcomes following single TBI, multiple TBI, and moderate and severe TBI. Given that in CTE we are really interested in RHI, and most of our cases have come from the setting of contact sports, I think it is most relevant to review the literature on contact sport athletes. *APOE* has been shown to confer unfavorable outcomes following exposure to contact sports as well. In 1997, Jordan et al.[5] looked at a small sample of current and former boxers and found that ε4 carriers were more impaired on a global function scale. In 2000, in a study of 53 active American professional football players, ε4 carriers were more impaired on measures of global cognition, processing speed, and attention.[6]

Dr. Stern also published in 2013[7] from our cohort on 68 pathologically proven cases of CTE without other neurodegenerative diseases. ε4 homozygotes were overrepresented in comparison to the overall population, but ε4 carriers did not differ in comparison to the overall population. The brain bank has grown substantially since this publication, so we are actively looking to replicate and expand on it. It is important to note that ε4 differs substantially across different ethnic backgrounds, so it is really important to consider that carefully when you are conducting analyses.

MAPT Haplotype

The microtubule associated protein tau (*MAPT*) haplotype is also important to consider in CTE. *MAPT* encodes the tau protein that we see in neurofibrillary tangles in CTE, as well as in Alzheimer's disease and several other neurodegenerative diseases. Rare mutations in *MAPT* cause an autosomal dominant tauopathy (FTDP-17) that takes on several clinical and neuropathological phenotypes that have been well described in the literature, including frontotemporal dementia, language and behavioral syndromes, parkinsonism, an amnestic syndrome, progressive supranuclear palsy (PSP), and corticobasal degeneration (CBD). Most likely, these rare mutations found in families are not causing CTE. There is a more common *MAPT* haplotype that has also been associated with other tauopathies that could be important.

When several SNPs are inherited together from a single parent, they are called a haplotype. In the setting of *MAPT*, there are two haplotypes, H1 and H2, that define two discrete alleles. H1 is defined by a region of complete linkage disequilibrium spanning the entire coding sequence and a much larger 900-kb region. H2 differs from H1 by a 238-base-pair deletion upstream of exon 10. The H2 haplotype is found in 20% to 30% of those with European ancestry, but it is absent or very rare in non-European populations. The are several H1 subhaplotypes identified on the H1 background. The H1 haplotype and H1 subhaplotypes have been implicated in various tauopathies, such as Alzheimer's disease, PSP, CBD, and primarily age-related tauopathy.[8] The tau protein has six major isoforms that result from alternative splicing of exons 2, 3, and 10. The splicing out or in of exon 10 results in isoforms with either three or four microtubule binding repeats (termed 3R or 4R). Several of the primary tauopathies, but not AD, have an excess of either the 3R or the 4R isoform. The *MAPT* H1 haplotype and subhaplotypes may alter the 3R:4R ratio. We are actively investigating whether *MAPT* haplotypes and subhaplotypes are associated with CTE pathology and if we see differences in the 3R:4R ratio in our CTE brains (Fig. 7.5).

FUTURE DIRECTIONS

We have a lot of plans for genetic studies of CTE. There are several cohorts that we plan to include in these analyses. The Veterans Affairs-Boston University-Concussion Legacy Foundation (VA-BU-CLF) brain bank has 225 neuropathologically confirmed cases and 75 neuropathologically confirmed controls, and we are adding more continuously. From the LEGEND (Longitudinal Examination to Gather Evidence of Neurodegenerative Disease) study, we have 75 cognitively normal clinical controls with known exposure, and from the DETECT (Diagnosing and Evaluating Traumatic Encephalopathy Using Clinical Tests) study, we have 95 former NFL players with rich endophenotype data. Dr. Stern told you about DIAGNOSE (Diagnostics, Imaging, and Genetics Network for the Objective Study and Evaluation) CTE (Chapter 3). We are actively recruiting 180 former NFL and college football players for whom we will also have rich clinical endophenotypes. We are also turning to the Alzheimer's Disease Genetic Consortium where we have more than we need of cognitively normal controls, but with unknown exposure. In these cohorts, we are taking multiple approaches. Initially, we have pursued a candidate gene approach, looking at *APOE* and *MAPT*, as well as with several other candidates that have been associated with other tauopathies. We will be conducting genome-wide genotyping on the full brain bank. We are also funded to conduct targeted deep sequencing of candidate genes that we hope will be informed by the genome-wide analysis.

ETHICS OF GENETIC TESTING

Traditionally, genetic testing has been limited to rare diseases with Mendelian inheritance patterns. In these diseases, having a mutation is largely deterministic: If you have the mutation, you will get the disease (with some caveats). Genetic susceptibility testing for common diseases with complex inheritance patterns is not nearly as straightforward because it is not deterministic but rather only provides information about risk. For instance, in Alzheimer's disease, having one copy of the *APOE* ε4 allele increases your odds of developing AD by two to three times, but having the allele does not mean you will develop the disease. Typically, genetic susceptibility testing is limited to risk variants that have a strong predictive value and to diseases for which medical decision making will be guided by knowledge of the genetic risk. For CTE, a disease that most likely will have a complex inheritance pattern, if we were to identify a risk variant with a strong predictive value, it very well could guide medical decision making because medical professionals could recommend that an individual refrain from engaging in contact sports. Genetic testing in CTE becomes stickier because that recommendation would probably have to come when an individual is still a minor. Genetic testing in minors is complicated by minors' capacity to consent and to really understand the possible implications of testing. Typically, genetic testing in minors only occurs when there is a family history, which may not be relevant for CTE, but certainly would sometimes be the case. Genetic testing for minors is usually only recommended

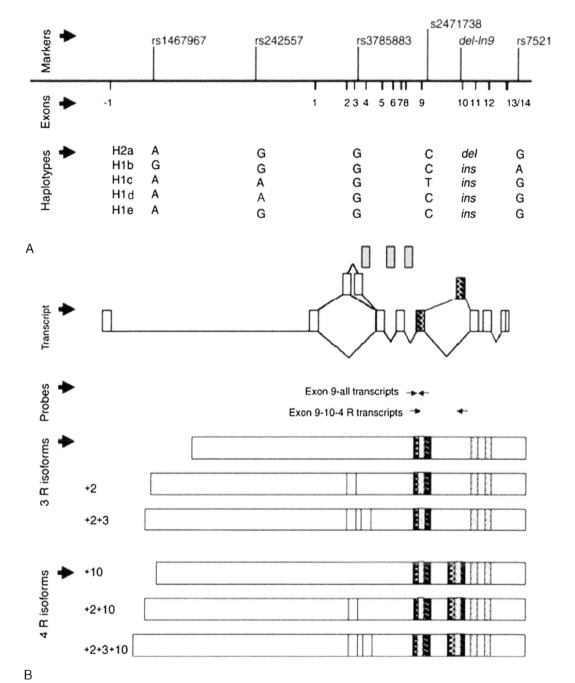

FIG. 7.5 (A) Shown are the locations of single-nucleotide polymorphisms (SNPs) used to define the four major *MAPT* haplotypes. Under the location of each SNP, the allele for that particular SNP is shown for each haplotype (e.g., for haplotype H2a: rs1467967=A, rs242557=G, rs3785883=G, rs2471738=C, del-In9=del, and rs7521=G). The del-In9 polymorphism tags all H1 haplotypes, separating them from H2. **(B)** Shown are the *MAPT* transcript and alternate splice isoforms. Stippled regions within the isoforms indicate the microtubule repeat regions. Isoforms containing exon 10 contain four microtubule-binding repeats (4R isoforms), and isoforms lacking exon 10 contain three microtubule-binding repeats (3R isoforms). (Adapted from Myers AJ, Pittman AM, Zhao AS, et al. The MAPT H1c risk haplotype is associated with increased expression of tau and especially of 4 repeat containing transcripts. *Neurobiology of Disease.* 2007;25(3):561–570. http://dx.doi.org/10.1016/j.nbd.2006.10.018.)

when medical decision making would occur during childhood, which would be the case for CTE. Genetic testing is also complicated by the need for a professional with genetic expertise. There are several million youths playing football in the United States, and typically their primary care providers do not have the time or the genetic expertise to counsel appropriately. The situation is further complicated by direct-to-consumer personal genomics testing companies that argue that the medical community is being paternalistic by advocating guidelines like the ones I've just mentioned. This topic could be a talk unto itself. The larger point is that even if we were able to find a genetic risk factor for CTE with a large effect size, we would still face several hurdles surrounding genetic testing.

CONCLUDING REMARKS

I hope that I've convinced you that the genetics of CTE is fascinating but complicated. As I stated at the beginning, I hope that we will continue having this course and that in the future, when I give this talk, it will focus less on what we have planned and more on what we know. Thank you to the organizers for inviting me to speak.

REFERENCES

1. Mez J, Solomon TM, Daneshvar DH, Stein TD, McKee AC. Pathologically confirmed chronic traumatic encephalopathy in a 25-year-old former college football player. *JAMA Neurology.* 2016 Mar;73(3):353–355. http://dx.doi.org/10.1001/jamaneurol.2015.3998. PMID: 26747562.
2. Montenigro PH, Alosco ML, Martin B, et al. Cumulative head impact exposure predicts later-life depression, apathy, executive dysfunction, and cognitive impairment in former high school and college football players. *Journal of Neurotrauma.* January 2016. http://online.liebertpub.com/doi/abs/10.1089/neu.2016.4413.
3. McGowan PO, Sasaki A, D'Alessio AC, et al. Epigenetic regulation of the glucocorticoid receptor in human brain associates with childhood abuse. *Nature Neuroscience.* 2009;12(3):342–348. http://dx.doi.org/10.1038/nn.2270.
4. Mayeux R, Ottman R, Maestre G, et al. Synergistic effects of traumatic head injury and apolipoprotein-epsilon 4 in patients with Alzheimer's disease. *Neurology.* 1995;45(3 Pt 1):555–557.
5. Jordan BD, Relkin NR, Ravdin LD, Jacobs AR, Bennett A, Gandy S. Apolipoprotein E epsilon4 associated with chronic traumatic brain injury in boxing. *JAMA.* 1997;278(2):136–140.
6. Kutner KC, Erlanger DM, Tsai J, Jordan B, Relkin NR. Lower cognitive performance of older football players possessing apolipoprotein E epsilon4. *Neurosurgery.* 2000;47(3):651–657. Discussion 657–658.
7. Stern RA, Daneshvar DH, Baugh CM, et al. Clinical presentation of chronic traumatic encephalopathy. *Neurology.* 2013;81(13):1122–1129. http://dx.doi.org/10.1212/WNL.0b013e3182a55f7f.
8. Myers AJ, Pittman AM, Zhao AS, et al. The MAPT H1c risk haplotype is associated with increased expression of tau and especially of 4 repeat containing transcripts. *Neurobiology of Disease.* 2007;25(3):561–570. http://dx.doi.org/10.1016/j.nbd.2006.10.018.
9. Idaghdour Y, Awadalla P. Exploiting gene expression variation to capture gene-environment interactions for disease. *Frontiers in Genetics.* 2013:3. http://dx.doi.org/10.3389/fgene.2012.00228.
10. Stein TD, Alvarez VE, McKee AC. Chronic traumatic encephalopathy: a spectrum of neuropathological changes following repetitive brain trauma in athletes and military personnel.. *Alzheimers Res Ther.* 2014;6(1):4. http://dx.doi.org/10.1186/alzrt234.

FURTHER READING

Gandy S, Dekosky ST. APOE ε4 status and traumatic brain injury on the gridiron or the battlefield. *Science Translational Medicine.* 2012;4(134):134ed4. http://dx.doi.org/10.1126/scitranslmed.3004274.

CHAPTER 8

Comorbid Pathology in Chronic Traumatic Encephalopathy

THOR D. STEIN

OVERVIEW OF COMORBID PATHOLOGIES SEEN IN CHRONIC TRAUMATIC ENCEPHALOPATHY

Chronic traumatic encephalopathy (CTE) is defined by a characteristic pattern of tau pathology that occurs within neurons, glia, and processes in a patchy distribution at the sulcal depths and around blood vessels[1] (Chapter 2). However, like many neurodegenerative diseases, CTE is also often associated with comorbid pathologies.

In our experience examining the group of individuals who have come to the Boston University-Veterans Affairs-Concussion Legacy Foundation (BU-VA-CLF) brain bank and developed CTE, we find that a slim majority of subjects with CTE (52%) do not have comorbid disease (Fig. 8.1). Many of these subjects are particularly young. However, despite the overall young age of this cohort compared to other brain banks, 48% do have comorbid disease, the most common of which is Alzheimer's disease (AD, 18%). The second most common comorbid pathology is Lewy body disease (16%), either with or without the clinical manifestation of Parkinson's disease or parkinsonism. About 9% have motor neuron disease/amyotrophic lateral sclerosis (ALS). An additional 6% have frontotemporal lobar degeneration (FTLD) that is often progressive supranuclear palsy or FTLD-TDP.

It is instructive to compare the frequency of comorbidity in CTE to what we see in AD. In over 300 cases from the BU Alzheimer Disease Center we see that half of subjects have AD without comorbid pathology (Fig. 8.2). In the subjects with comorbid disease, the majority of them have Lewy body disease (43% of total). A similar percentage as in CTE has comorbid FTLD (6%). Some of the AD subjects also had CTE (2%). None had ALS, which is the biggest difference between the subjects with CTE, where 9% had comorbid motor neuron disease.

COMPARISON OF PROGRESSION OF TAU PATHOLOGY IN CTE AND AD

Alzheimer's disease is the most frequent comorbidity in CTE. In order to distinguish the putative progression of CTE from AD, it is instructive to look at the stages of CTE as they have been defined and compare them to the stages of AD. As shown in Fig. 8.3, in CTE the abnormal accumulation of hyperphosphorylated tau first appears in the neocortex and locus coeruleus (CTE stage I), then involves the diencephalon (CTE stage II), next the medial temporal lobe (CTE stage III), and finally widespread involvement of neocortical, brainstem, and cerebellar regions (CTE stage IV). This apparent top-down progression in CTE is in contrast to the bottom-up progression in AD where the tau pathology first occurs in the brainstem (Braak stages a to c), next involves the entorhinal cortex (stages 1a, 1b, I-II), then more widespread involvement of the medial temporal lobe (stages III-IV), and finally widespread involvement of the neocortex (stages V-VI).

β-AMYLOID IN CTE

Although β-amyloid (Aβ) is not a defining feature of CTE, it is the most frequent comorbid pathology and may play a role in disease progression when these pathologies co-occur. Therefore, we set out to determine the role of Aβ in CTE.[2] Specifically, we tested whether Aβ plaque deposition is altered in CTE compared to AD, whether it occurs more frequently in CTE, and whether the presence of Aβ worsens the tau pathology and clinical outcomes in CTE. To do that, we examined our cohort of individuals with CTE in the brain bank at the time, which was 114 cases. These were athletes from a variety of sports but predominantly American football and they played at the professional or the collegiate level; some were military veterans who were exposed to blast and concussive injury during

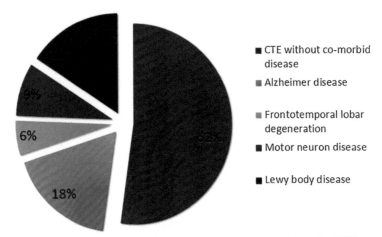

FIG. 8.1 Comorbid disease in chronic traumatic encephalopathy (CTE).

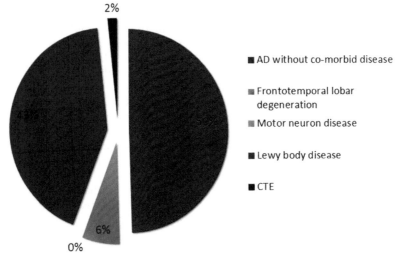

FIG. 8.2 Comorbid disease in Alzheimer's disease (AD).

combat. We divided the cohort into different pathological groups, CTE without Aβ and CTE with Aβ, and compared them to a group of subjects with AD (Table 8.1). Looking at CTE overall the average age was 60, which is young for a neurodegenerative cohort. Nevertheless, 52% of them had diffuse plaques, and just over a third of them had neuritic plaques, a more mature, dense core plaque that is associated with tau-positive neurites. When the subject groups are examined by CTE stage, plaque deposition increases with stage and age: at stage 1 CTE with an average age of 35, 15% of individuals with CTE have diffuse plaques and none have neuritic plaques; at stage 2, one-third of subjects have diffuse plaques and 20% have neuritic plaques; at stage 3, 44% have diffuse plaques and 27% have neuritic

plaques; finally at stage 4, the average age of subjects is in their 70s, and 87% of them have diffuse plaques and 70% have neuritic plaques. Thus, stage IV CTE has a similar frequency of plaque deposition as AD, where 84% have diffuse plaques and all subjects have neuritic plaques, as it is part of the definition of the disease.

Next we examined demographic and exposure associations between groups (Table 8.2). There was no significant difference in the amount of years played in contact sports between the CTE subjects with or without Aβ. There was an increase in concussions such that CTE subjects with Aβ had more concussions but the difference was not significant likely due to the variability in concussion reporting. In CTE subjects with Aβ, the average age of death is more than 20 years greater than

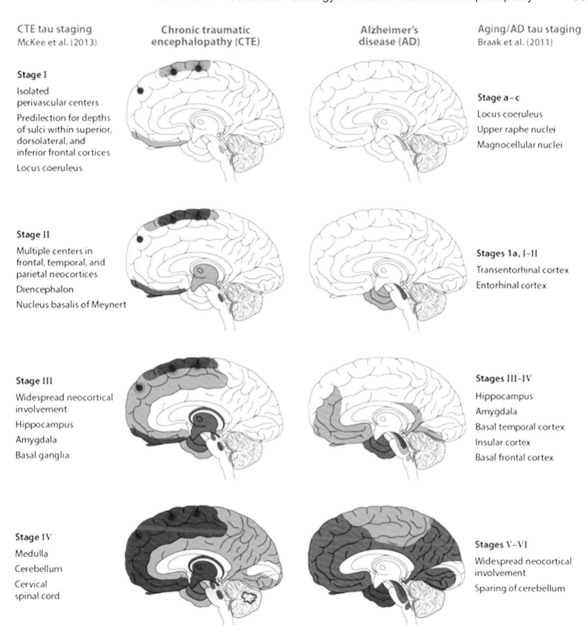

CTE tau staging McKee et al. (2013)	Chronic traumatic encephalopathy (CTE)	Alzheimer's disease (AD)	Aging/AD tau staging Braak et al. (2011)
Stage I Isolated perivascular centers Predilection for depths of sulci within superior, dorsolateral, and inferior frontal cortices Locus coeruleus			**Stage a–c** Locus coeruleus Upper raphe nuclei Magnocellular nuclei
Stage II Multiple centers in frontal, temporal, and parietal neocortices Diencephalon Nucleus basalis of Meynert			**Stages 1a, I–II** Transentorhinal cortex Entorhinal cortex
Stage III Widespread neocortical involvement Hippocampus Amygdala Basal ganglia			**Stages III–IV** Hippocampus Amygdala Basal temporal cortex Insular cortex Basal frontal cortex
Stage IV Medulla Cerebellum Cervical spinal cord			**Stages V–VI** Widespread neocortical involvement Sparing of cerebellum

FIG. 8.3 Comparison of hyperphosphorylated tau progression in chronic traumatic encephalopathy and Alzheimer's disease. (With permission from Montenigro, et al. *Annual Review of Clinical Psychology*;11.)

subjects without Aβ. The age of symptom onset was also increased in CTE subjects with Aβ by about 20 years.

Age-Dependent Aβ Deposition

Clearly, Aβ deposition is an age-dependent process. However, it is unknown whether the frequency or the pattern of Aβ deposition in CTE is different from

what would be expected in the general population. To attempt to address this, we compared our results to a prior study that looked at over 2300 subjects from a hospital autopsy service in Germany[3] (Fig. 8.4). They found a clear age-dependent increase in Aβ in the brain such that no one under the age of 40 had Aβ (unless they had Down's syndrome). For individuals in their 40s,

TABLE 8.1
Frequency of Aβ Deposition in CTE

	n	Mean age at death (year)	DP Frequency (%)	NP Frequency (%)
CTE (all)	114	60	52	36
Stage I	13	35	15	0
Stage II	30	52	33	20
Stage III	34	62	44	27
Stage IV	37	75	87	70
AD	319	80	84	100

Aβ, β-amyloid; AD, Alzheimer's disease; CTE, chronic traumatic encephalopathy; DP, diffuse plaque; NP, neuritic plaque.
With permission from Stein TD, Montenigro PH, Alvarez VE, Xia W, Crary JF, Tripodis Y, et al. Beta-amyloid deposition in chronic traumatic encephalopathy. Acta Neuropathologica. July 2015;130(1):21–34. PMCID: 4529056.

TABLE 8.2
Age Is Associated With Aβ Plaques

	n	CTE Mean±SEM	n	CTE with Aβ Mean±SEM	P-Value*
Age at death (year)	55	48.2±2.6	59	71.6±1.4	**<0.001**
Athletic exposure (year)	51	15.0±1.0	46	15.9±0.9	0.500
Number of concussions	48	11.5±3.0	41	24.2±6.6	0.071
Age at Sx onset (year)	43	36.2±2.3	42	54.2±2.3	**<0.001**

*Student's t test; significant P values are in bold.
Aβ, β-amyloid; CTE, chronic traumatic encephalopathy; Sx, symptom.
With permission from Stein TD, Montenigro PH, Alvarez VE, Xia W, Crary JF, Tripodis Y, et al. Beta-amyloid deposition in chronic traumatic encephalopathy. Acta Neuropathologica. July 2015;130(1):21–34. PMCID: 4529056.

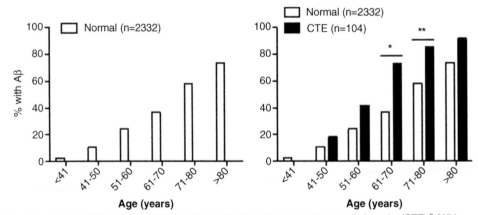

FIG. 8.4 β-amyloid (Aβ) deposition is accelerated in chronic traumatic encephalopathy (CTE).[3] (With permission from Stein TD, Montenigro PH, Alvarez VE, Xia W, Crary JF, Tripodis Y, et al. Beta-amyloid deposition in chronic traumatic encephalopathy. Acta Neuropathologica. July 2015;130(1):21–34. PMCID: 4529056.)

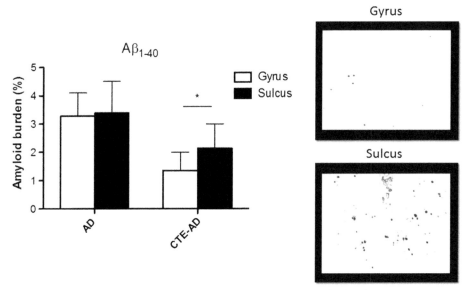

FIG. 8.5 β-amyloid (Aβ) burden is greater in the sulcus than in the gyrus in chronic traumatic encephalopathy (CTE)-Alzheimer's disease (AD). (With permission from Stein TD, Montenigro PH, Alvarez VE, Xia W, Crary JF, Tripodis Y, et al. Beta-amyloid deposition in chronic traumatic encephalopathy. *Acta Neuropathologica*. July 2015;130(1):21–34. PMCID: 4529056.)

about 10% had some Aβ deposition, and this frequency steadily increased to decade age 80 where it plateaued at 80%. This plateau suggests that there are about 20% of individuals who are resistant to developing amyloid in the brain no matter their age. In CTE we first see amyloid in the brain in subjects in their 40s, where it is already increased compared to the normal autopsy cohort. The frequency of Aβ deposition continues to increase with decade age and is nearly 80% in CTE subjects in their 60s. This is almost as high as what is seen in the normal autopsy cohort in their 80s, suggesting that there is a 15- to 20-year acceleration of Aβ deposition in subjects with CTE. The frequency of Aβ deposition continues to increase such that it reaches almost 90% for subjects in their 80s, suggesting that people otherwise resistant will eventually accumulate Aβ if they have CTE or perhaps exposure to repetitive head impacts.

We next examined the pattern of Aβ deposition to determine if there were differences in how Aβ is deposited in CTE compared to AD. The striking spatial pattern of tau pathology present within sulcal depths in CTE suggests that Aβ deposition might also be concentrated there. This pattern may be due to axonal or other cellular damage from stress concentration of repetitive head impacts. Therefore, we quantified the number of plaques deposited at the gyral crest and compared that to the bottom third of the sulcus within the dorsolateral

frontal cortex. We found that in AD there is no difference in the burden of Aβ plaques within the gyrus or the sulcus. On the other hand, in CTE there is a significant increase in Aβ plaque deposition within the sulcus compared to the gyrus (Fig. 8.5). We looked biochemically to determine the kind of Aβ present and found that $A\beta_{1-40}$, and not $A\beta_{1-42}$, was significantly increased in the sulcus compared to the gyrus (Fig. 8.6). Interestingly, $A\beta_{1-40}$ is one of the major components in cerebral amyloid angiopathy, which we also see within many of the CTE subjects within the sulcal depths. In addition, $A\beta_{1-40}$ is a major component of neuritic plaques, which are associated with tau pathology.

Association of Aβ With CTE Stage and Tauopathy

We next tested the hypothesis that Aβ is associated with worse tau pathology in CTE. CTE subjects with Aβ (Consortium to Establish a Registry of Alzheimer's disease [CERAD] pathology stage >0) had a significantly greater median CTE stage when compared to subjects without Aβ (CERAD stage = 0; Fig. 8.7). When subjects were grouped by decade age of death to eliminate the age difference between groups, we found that CTE subjects with Aβ in their 60s had a significantly increased CTE stage compared to those without Aβ. Biochemical analysis of an early tau phosphorylation site present

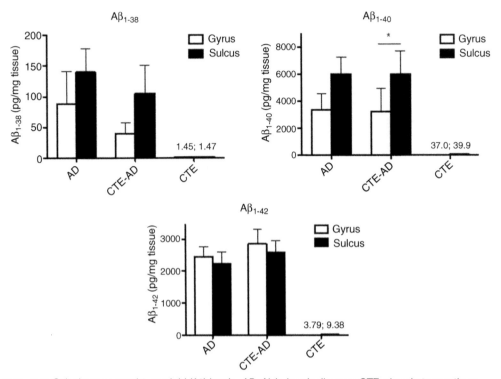

FIG. 8.6 Sulcal versus gyral β-amyloid (Aβ) levels. *AD*, Alzheimer's disease; *CTE*, chronic traumatic encephalopathy. (With permission from Stein TD, Montenigro PH, Alvarez VE, Xia W, Crary JF, Tripodis Y, et al. Beta-amyloid deposition in chronic traumatic encephalopathy. *Acta Neuropathologica*. July 2015;130(1): 21–34. PMCID: 4529056.)

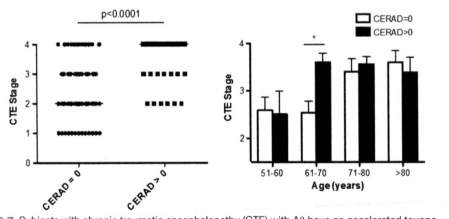

FIG. 8.7 Subjects with chronic traumatic encephalopathy (CTE) with Aβ have an accelerated tauopathy. *CERAD*, Consortium to Establish a Registry of Alzheimer's Disease. (With permission from Stein TD, Montenigro PH, Alvarez VE, Xia W, Crary JF, Tripodis Y, et al. Beta-amyloid deposition in chronic traumatic encephalopathy. *Acta Neuropathologica*. July 2015;130(1):21–34. PMCID: 4529056.)

in AD (ptau231) showed that the presence of neuritic plaques was associated with increased ptau231 levels in CTE, but that levels were still greatest in AD or in subjects with both CTE and AD (Fig. 8.8). Thus, ptau231 appears to be a phosphorylation site that is largely driven by Aβ pathology in CTE.

Association of Aβ With Dementia and Parkinsonism

Examination of clinical outcomes found that almost 90% of subjects with CTE and Aβ experienced CTE symptoms before death compared to 76% of CTE without Aβ subjects, although this difference was not quite significant (Table 8.3). There was a significant increase in the frequency of dementia in the presence of Aβ though: the percentage of subjects diagnosed with dementia in life by a physician increased from 20% in

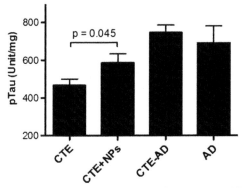

FIG. 8.8 Levels of ptau231 in middle frontal gyrus. *AD*, Alzheimer's disease; *CTE*, chronic traumatic encephalopathy; *NP*, neuritic plaque. (With permission from Stein TD, Montenigro PH, Alvarez VE, Xia W, Crary JF, Tripodis Y, et al. Beta-amyloid deposition in chronic traumatic encephalopathy. *Acta Neuropathologica*. July 2015;130(1):21–34. PMCID: 4529056.)

CTE alone to 73% in CTE with Aβ, and this difference was significant when controlling for age. The frequency of the symptoms of Parkinson's disease (parkinsonism) also increased from 2% to 25% in the presence of Aβ and was significant controlling for age. Perhaps underlying this increase in parkinsonism was a similar significant increase in the frequency of pathological Lewy body disease with Aβ in CTE.

MODELING THE PATHOLOGY

As we have seen, Aβ, tau, and Lewy body pathologies occur later in life, sometimes decades after cessation of repetitive head impact exposure. Recently, we sought to determine some of the earliest changes occurring in the brain in order to start to develop models of disease progression. One of the earliest changes following brain injury is the activation of inflammatory cells. Therefore, we looked at the density of activated microglia identified with a CD68 immunostain within the dorsolateral frontal cortex compared to the development of tau pathology and dementia in American football players over time.[4] The regression models of these results are superimposed and plotted in Fig. 8.9 as a function of time defined as the number of years from first exposure to death. The assumption here is that some injury occurs from the very first time one begins playing football; acutely the brain may recover, but chronic exposure to repetitive head impacts may eventually lead to disease. In fact, we found that there was elevated density of activated microglia in the frontal cortex of CTE in even the youngest subjects and that the density of these cells slowly, but significantly, increased over time. In contrast, tau pathology occurred many years after the first exposure to football play and increased at a much steeper rate. Once this tau pathology reached a threshold about 30 to 40 years after

TABLE 8.3
Aβ Is Associated With Dementia, Parkinsonism, and LBD Pathology in CTE

	CTE Frequency (%) (+/−)	CTE with Aβ Frequency (%) (+/−)	P-Value[a]	P-Value[b]
CTE Sx	76 (37/12)	90 (43/5)	0.059	0.419
Dementia	20 (10/39)	73 (35/13)	**<0.001**	**0.013**
Parkinsonism	2.1 (1/48)	25 (12/36)	**0.001**	**0.050**
LBD pathology	3.7 (2/52)	35 (19/35)	**<0.001**	**0.019**

Aβ, β-amyloid; *CTE*, chronic traumatic encephalopathy; *LBD*, Lewy body disease; *Sx*, symptom.
[a]Pearson χ² test.
[b]Logistic regression controlling for age; significant P values are in bold.
With permission from Stein TD, Montenigro PH, Alvarez VE, Xia W, Crary JF, Tripodis Y, et al. Beta-amyloid deposition in chronic traumatic encephalopathy. *Acta Neuropathologica*. July 2015;130(1):21–34. PMCID: 4529056.

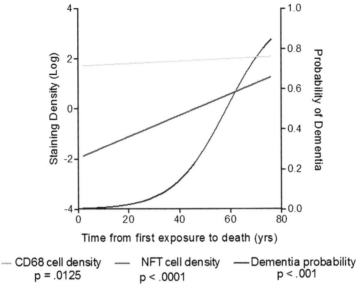

— CD68 cell density   — NFT cell density   —Dementia probability
p = .0125   p < .0001   p < .001

FIG. 8.9 Progression of neuroinflammation, tau pathology, and development of dementia in chronic traumatic encephalopathy. (With permission from Cherry JD, Tripodis Y, Alvarez VE, Huber B, Kiernan PT, Daneshvar DH, et al. Microglial neuroinflammation contributes to tau accumulation in chronic traumatic encephalopathy. *Acta Neuropathologica Communications*. October 28, 2016;4(1):112. PMCID: 5084333.)

the first exposure, there was a sudden increase in the probability of developing dementia (Fig. 8.9). Overall, these data suggest a temporal sequence in CTE, where first microglia are activated, then tau pathology develops, and subsequently subjects become demented. In order to test these pathological associations we developed a statistical model using two simultaneous linear regressions to test the effects of the two independent variables (1) age and (2) years of exposure to football play on the outcome variables (1) density of activated microglia and (2) tau pathology. This simultaneous equation regression model incorporates a possible feedback mechanism between microglial activation and tau pathology. In fact, previous work in AD using animal and in vitro models has shown that activated microglia can drive tau pathology and that tau pathology can also lead to the activation of microglia in a potential feed-forward mechanism.[5,6] When we modeled this pathology in our cohort of football players and controls not exposed to contact sports, we found that the number of years of exposure to football play was significantly associated with the development of tau pathology both directly and via increased microglia. Increased age was also significantly associated with tau pathology but had no significant effect on microglial activation. Supporting the concept of a feedback loop, increased microglial activation led to increased

tau pathology, and increased tau pathology had a smaller, but significant, positive effect on microglial activation. Fig. 8.10 is a visual representation of these results, where the significant interactions are indicated with arrows and the length of the arrows are roughly proportionate to the effect size. Going forward, we need to build and refine this model to determine how the other comorbid pathologies that occur with age and CTE, including Aβ, Lewy bodies, and TDP-43, might interact with neuroinflammation and tau pathology and potentially be driven by age and exposure to repetitive head impacts.

CONCLUSIONS

Overall, the early presence of comorbid pathology in CTE suggests that some aging processes are accelerated. In particular, Aβ deposition was altered and accelerated in CTE compared to a normal aging cohort. Moreover, Aβ was associated with worse pathology and poor clinical outcomes in CTE even when controlling for age. Thus, identification of comorbid pathology will be important in predicting disease course. The interpretation of blood and cerebrospinal fluid biomarkers and positron emission tomography neuroimaging using both amyloid and tau ligands will need to consider the possibility of Aβ pathology in persons older

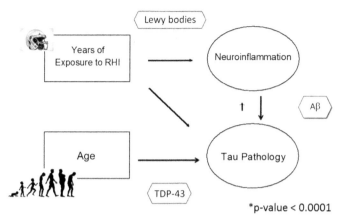

FIG. 8.10 Modeling the pathology.

than 40 with CTE. In addition, motor neuron disease is a frequent comorbidity in CTE, and further research probing potential common mechanisms is required. Finally, one of the earliest changes found to occur following contact sports exposure is microglial activation in the frontal cortex, and over time this inflammatory response may contribute to the development of tau pathology in CTE. Overall, the development of biomarkers and strategies to interfere with disease pathogenesis requires a detailed understanding of pathological mechanisms in CTE.

REFERENCES

1. McKee AC, Cairns NJ, Dickson DW, Folkerth RD, Keene CD, Litvan I, et al. The first NINDS/NIBIB consensus meeting to define neuropathological criteria for the diagnosis of chronic traumatic encephalopathy. *Acta Neuropathologica*. January 2016;131(1):75–86. PMCID: 4698281.

2. Stein TD, Montenigro PH, Alvarez VE, Xia W, Crary JF, Tripodis Y, et al. Beta-amyloid deposition in chronic traumatic encephalopathy. *Acta Neuropathologica*. July 2015;130(1):21–34. PMCID: 4529056.

3. Braak H, Thal DR, Ghebremedhin E, Del Tredici K. Stages of the pathologic process in Alzheimer disease: age categories from 1 to 100 years. *Journal of Neuropathology and Experimental neurology*. November 2011;70(11):960–969.

4. Cherry JD, Tripodis Y, Alvarez VE, Huber B, Kiernan PT, Daneshvar DH, et al. Microglial neuroinflammation contributes to tau accumulation in chronic traumatic encephalopathy. *Acta Neuropathologica Communications*. October 28, 2016;4(1):112. PMCID: 5084333.

5. Bhaskar K, Konerth M, Kokiko-Cochran ON, Cardona A, Ransohoff RM, Lamb BT. Regulation of tau pathology by the microglial fractalkine receptor. *Neuron*. October 6, 2010;68(1):19–31. PMCID: 2950825.

6. Maphis N, Xu G, Kokiko-Cochran ON, Cardona AE, Ransohoff RM, Lamb BT, et al. Loss of tau rescues inflammation-mediated neurodegeneration. *Frontiers in Neuroscience*. 2015;9:196. PMCID: 4452825.

CHAPTER 9

Differential Diagnosis and Treatment of Chronic Traumatic Encephalopathy

ANDREW E. BUDSON

INTRODUCTION

What I would like to talk about this morning is how you can recognize and treat an individual with chronic traumatic encephalopathy (CTE) when they walk into your clinic. So this talk is specifically for all the clinicians in the audience. I will discuss in some detail the most common neurological degenerative disorder that you're going to see in your clinic, and that is Alzheimer's disease. We are then going to contrast Alzheimer's disease with other disorders. How are they each different from Alzheimer's? And, of course, we are going to end off the talk focusing on CTE and how you can distinguish CTE from these other disorders, including vascular dementia, dementia with Lewy bodies, and frontotemporal dementia. If you want to learn more about these other disorders in detail, see Ref. 1.

ALZHEIMER'S DISEASE IS THE MOST COMMON CAUSE OF DEMENTIA

Dementia increases geometrically with age. It is present in 5% to 10% of individuals over the age of 65 and in about 50% of those over the age of 85. One of the points that I want to bring home in my talk is that Alzheimer's disease is by far the most common cause of dementia, about 70% if you consider it not only by itself, but also when it is present in combination with other disorders such as cerebrovascular disease or Lewy body disease.

Diagnosis of Alzheimer's Disease Dementia

I would like to start with a case example. It's an 81-year-old man who came in with memory difficulties. His family said it had started about 8 years ago when he got lost, even on the familiar route to his son's house. He also began asking the same questions again and again and *again*, driving everyone a bit crazy. Things gradually became worse over the past 8 years. For the last 6 to 12 months, he couldn't remember any

new information whatsoever. For example, he had a new grandchild born in the family. In addition to not being able to remember the grandchild's name, which was unusual in itself, he also couldn't even remember the fact that he had a new grandchild. That's when his family realized that this problem must be more than normal aging. He also had a lot of word-finding difficulties. Interestingly, he could still remember his days during World War II, and his family noted that his memory was quite good for those early days. So, this story is a fairly classic history for Alzheimer's disease, as most of you probably know.

Check vitamin D along with B12 and thyroid function

I would like to mention one of the new things that I am now thinking about when I see a patient like this one in the clinic, and that is to either check vitamin D levels or to simply recommend that my patients take vitamin D3 2000 IU daily. Low levels of vitamin D have not been shown in a mechanistic way to increase the incidence of dementia, but I was impressed by this paper from the journal *Neurology* in 2014 (Fig. 9.1). If we look at the years of follow-up on the x-axis and the percent who develop dementia on the y-axis, you can see that as the serum levels of vitamin D go from being sufficient to deficient to severely deficient, the incidence of dementia goes up dramatically.[2] So, I do recommend that you check the vitamin D levels along with the B12 and thyroid stimulating hormone when you are thinking about laboratory blood tests to get for your patients with possible dementia.

Criteria for dementia and major neurocognitive disorder

Let's talk about the criteria for dementia (Box 9.1).[3] These are the National Institute on Aging—Alzheimer's Association criteria that will classify any type of dementia, including dementia from CTE or from the

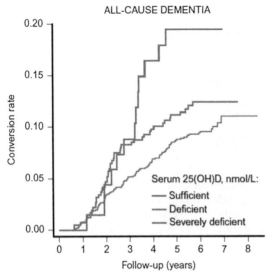

FIG. 9.1 Kaplan-Meier curves for unadjusted rates of all-cause dementia by serum 25-hydroxyvitamin D [25(OH)D] concentrations. (Adapted from Littlejohns TJ, Henley WE, Lang IA, et al. Vitamin D and the risk of dementia and Alzheimer disease. *Neurology*. 2014;83: 920–928.)

traumatic encephalopathy syndrome that Dr. Robert Stern described to you (Chapter 3). First, there must be a decline in the individual's function from his or her prior level. That is one of the core features of dementia. In addition, the functional decline must be caused by cognitive impairment. Knowledge of cognitive impairment can come from the patient or more commonly from the informant (usually a family member). There also must be some type of objective cognitive testing, whether it's done with a brief test in the office or by sending the patient for formal neuropsychological testing. Two or more cognitive domains need to be impaired. The Diagnostic and Statistical Manual of Mental Disorders, Fifth Edition (DSM-5), criteria for major neurocognitive disorder are very similar to those for dementia.

Criteria for Alzheimer's disease dementia

After we made the diagnosis of dementia using the criteria for dementia of any cause, the question is how do we diagnose Alzheimer's disease dementia in particular (Box 9.2).[3] For the National Institute on Aging—Alzheimer's Association criteria, patients first must meet the criteria for all-cause dementia that I just mentioned. There must be a slow, insidious onset over months

---

BOX 9.1
National Institute on Aging—Alzheimer's Association All-Cause Dementia Core Clinical Criteria

CLINICAL CRITERIA

1. Interfere with the ability to function at work or at usual activities; and
2. Represent a decline from previous levels of functioning and performing; and
3. Are not explained by delirium or major psychiatric disorder.
4. Cognitive impairment is detected and diagnosed through a combination of (1) history taking from the patient and a knowledgeable informant and (2) an objective cognitive assessment, either a "bedside" mental status examination or neuropsychological testing.
5. The cognitive or behavioral impairment involves a minimum of two of the following domains:
   a. Impaired ability to acquire and remember new information—symptoms include: repetitive questions or conversations, misplacing personal belongings, forgetting events or appointments, getting lost on a familiar route.

   b. Impaired reasoning and handling of complex tasks, poor judgment—symptoms include: poor understanding of safety risks, inability to manage finances, poor decision-making ability, inability to plan complex or sequential activities.

   c. Impaired visuospatial abilities—symptoms include: inability to recognize faces or common objects or to find objects in direct view despite good acuity, inability to operate simple implements, or orient clothing to the body.

   d. Impaired language functions (speaking, reading, writing)—symptoms include: difficulty thinking of common words while speaking, hesitations; speech, spelling, and writing errors.

   e. Changes in personality, behavior, or comportment—symptoms include: uncharacteristic mood fluctuations such as agitation, impaired motivation, initiative, apathy, loss of drive, social withdrawal, decreased interest in previous activities, loss of empathy, compulsive or obsessive behaviors, socially unacceptable behaviors.

Adapted from McKhann GM, Knopman DS, Chertkow H, et al. The diagnosis of dementia due to Alzheimer's disease: recommendations from the National Institute on Aging-Alzheimer's Association workgroups on diagnostic guidelines for Alzheimer's disease. *Alzheimer's and Dementia*. 2011;7:263–269.

BOX 9.2
National Institute on Aging—Alzheimer's Association (NIA-AA) Probable AD Dementia: Core Clinical Criteria

CORE CLINICAL CRITERIA
Probable AD Dementia is Diagnosed When the Patient

1. Meets NIA-AA criteria for dementia described in Box 9.1 and, in addition, has the following characteristics:

   a. Insidious onset. Symptoms have a gradual onset over months to years, not sudden over hours or days;

   b. Clear-cut history of worsening of cognition by report or observation; and

   c. The initial and most prominent cognitive deficits are evident on history and examination in one of the following categories:

      i. Amnestic presentation: It is the most common syndromic presentation of AD dementia. The deficits should include impairment in learning and recall of recently learned information. There should also be evidence of cognitive dysfunction in at least one other cognitive domain, as defined in the NIA-AA criteria for dementia described in Box 9.1.

      ii. Nonamnestic presentations:

         i. Language presentation: The most prominent deficits are in word finding, but deficits in other cognitive domains should be present.

         ii. Visuospatial presentation: The most prominent deficits are in spatial cognition, including object agnosia, impaired face recognition, simultanagnosia, and alexia. Deficits in other cognitive domains should be present.

         iii. Executive dysfunction: The most prominent deficits are impaired reasoning, judgment, and problem solving. Deficits in other cognitive domains should be present.

   d. The diagnosis of probable AD dementia should not be applied when there is evidence of (1) substantial concomitant cerebrovascular disease, defined by a history of a stroke temporally related to the onset or worsening of cognitive impairment; or the presence of multiple or extensive infarcts or severe white matter hyperintensity burden; or (2) core features of dementia with Lewy bodies other than dementia itself; or (3) prominent features of behavioral variant frontotemporal dementia; or (4) prominent features of semantic variant primary progressive aphasia or nonfluent/agrammatic variant primary progressive aphasia; or (5) evidence for another concurrent, active neurological disease, or a nonneurological medical comorbidity or use of medication that could have a substantial effect on cognition.

Adapted from McKhann GM, Knopman DS, Chertkow H, et al. The diagnosis of dementia due to Alzheimer's disease: recommendations from the National Institute on Aging-Alzheimer's Association workgroups on diagnostic guidelines for Alzheimer's disease. *Alzheimer's and Dementia*. 2011;7:263–269.

---

to years, and there needs to be progressive cognitive impairment. It is recognized that Alzheimer's disease dementia most commonly occurs with the amnestic or memory loss presentation, but that it sometimes presents in a nonamnestic presentation such as with language or word-finding problems, visuospatial problems, or executive dysfunction problems. The main exclusionary criteria are other causes of dementias, such as vascular dementia, dementia with Lewy bodies, frontotemporal, CTE, etc. Again, the DSM-5 criteria for major neurocognitive disorder due to Alzheimer's disease are very similar.

Biomarkers and the continuum of Alzheimer's disease

We now think about Alzheimer's disease as a continuum (Fig. 9.2).[4] It starts off in the preclinical phase before any symptoms are present. When the mild cognitive impairment (MCI) stage is present, it means that cognitive function has begun to slip, and we can pick that up on standardized pencil and paper tests. But because people with MCI work a little bit harder, they compensate for their cognitive impairment and they can still function normally. Finally, when function is impaired, we have the onset of dementia.

I am now going to talk about some biomarkers. This will be a brief introduction; you're going to hear a lot more about biomarkers throughout the rest of the course. If we look at Fig. 9.3, if we are going to be detecting Alzheimer's disease based on clinical function, that means that we are diagnosing it in the dementia stage. If we simply do paper and pencil tests, we can pick it up earlier, in the MCI stage. If we look at the brain structure with an MRI scan, we can pick it up even earlier, in the preclinical phase. If we look for injury to neurons that elevates levels of tau in the spinal fluid, we can pick it up earlier. If we look for synaptic dysfunction using, for example, a fluorodeoxyglucose (FDG) PET scan, we can see evidence of Alzheimer's disease earlier. Finally, if we look for evidence of abnormal β-amyloid in the spinal fluid or with a PET scan we can detect Alzheimer's even earlier.

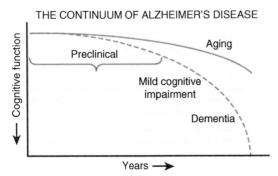

FIG. 9.2 The continuum of cognitive loss in normal aging and Alzheimer's disease. (Adapted from Sperling RA, Aisen PS, Beckett LA, et al. Toward defining the preclinical stages of Alzheimer's disease: recommendations from the National Institute on Aging—Alzheimer's Association workgroups on diagnostic guidelines for Alzheimer's disease. *Alzheimer's and Dementia*. 2011;7:280–292.)

Biomarkers in clinical practice

Let's talk a little bit about using some of these biomarkers in day-to-day clinical practice. A structural scan is, of course, very important in any type of workup for cognitive impairment. And what I am looking for is atrophy of the medial temporal lobes, anterior temporal lobes, and parietal cortices, as you can see in Fig. 9.4. Note that you don't have to do an MRI scan, here is a CT scan showing you that medial temporal lobe atrophy—the black spaces pointed at by the arrows are enlargements of the temporal horn of the lateral ventricle because of the shrinking of the hippocampus (Fig. 9.5). You'll hear more about MRI markers of disease from Dr. Martha Shenton (Chapter 11).

We can also look at the cerebrospinal fluid (CSF). For Alzheimer's disease, we are looking for a drop in β-amyloid and increase in phospho-tau, total tau, or both. Note that I don't perform this test routinely, but in an individual in whom it's very important to make a positive diagnosis (and not just rule out other things) or if the prognosis is important, this is one test that I may do. It is a particularly good test for a young patient with memory loss, say, younger than age 65. Because Alzheimer's disease is less common in young individuals, I would want to confirm my clinical diagnosis with such a test before I stopped looking for other possible causes of memory loss—such as CTE. One commercial lab that you can send CSF specimens to look for abnormal levels of β-amyloid

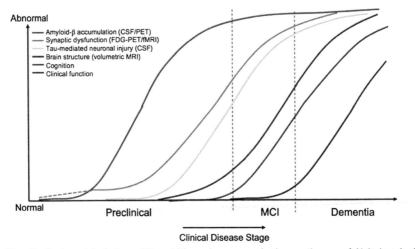

FIG. 9.3 Hypothetical model of when different biomarkers occur in the continuum of Alzheimer's disease, from preclinical to mild cognitive impairment (MCI) to dementia. (From Sperling RA, Aisen PS, Beckett LA, et al. Toward defining the preclinical stages of Alzheimer's disease: recommendations from the National Institute on Aging—Alzheimer's Association workgroups on diagnostic guidelines for Alzheimer's disease. *Alzheimer's and Dementia*. 2011;7:280–292.)

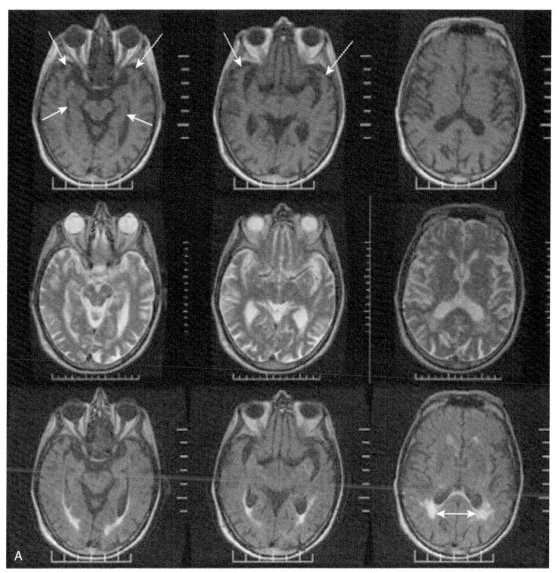

FIG. 9.4 Selected slices of an MRI scan of a patient with mild Alzheimer's disease. Panels (**A**) and (**B**) show the same six axial slices of brain from T1 (top), T2 (middle), and fluid-attenuated inversion recovery (FLAIR) (bottom) sequences. Panel (**C**) shows five T1 coronal slices and one T1 sagittal slice. The T1 images provide the best anatomical resolution, showing mild atrophy of the hippocampus (*thin solid arrows*), anterior temporal lobe (*thin dotted arrows*), and parietal cortex (*thick dotted arrows*). FLAIR images (in combination with T2) show vascular disease best (*double-headed arrow*). Note that the small vessel ischemic cerebrovascular disease shown here is average for an older adult. (From Budson AE, Solomon PR. *Memory Loss, Alzheimer's Disease, and Dementia: A Practical Guide for Clinicians*, 2nd ed. Elsevier; 2016.)

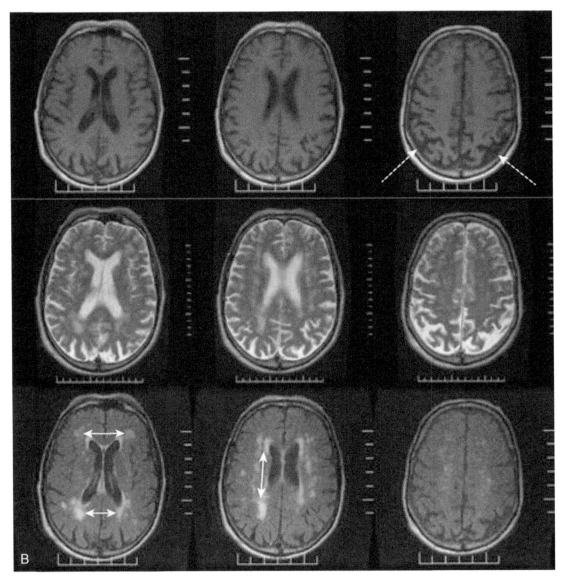

FIG. 9.4,   cont'd

and tau is Athena Diagnostics, www.athenadiagnostic s.com. You'll hear more about fluid biomarkers from Dr. Kaj Blennow (Chapter 10).

Another test that you can obtain is an FDG PET scan. Fig. 9.6 shows the brain metabolism revealed by an FDG PET scan in Alzheimer's disease. You can see decreased metabolism in the temporal lobes as well as in the parietal lobes. I use this study if the patient is clearly demented and I am not sure if it is Alzheimer's disease, CTE, frontotemporal dementia, or dementia

with Lewy bodies and figuring out the answer is going to be helpful in treating the patient. I am going to show some examples using FDG PET scans in other disorders as well.

The other thing that came up recently in the last couple of years is that we can also image β-amyloid in patients with Alzheimer's disease while they are still living. Fig. 9.7 shows an example with florbetapir (AMYViD), the first amyloid PET tracer approved by the US Food and Drug Administration (FDA) in

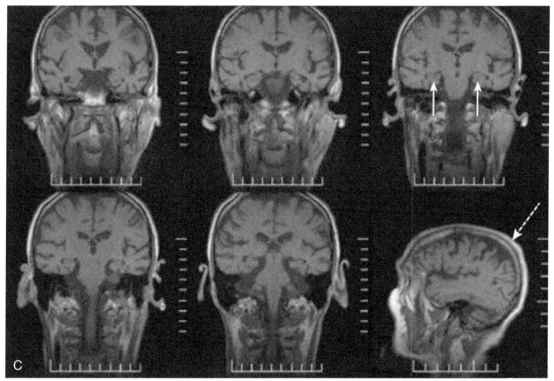

FIG. 9.4,   cont'd

2012. There are also two other tracers that are FDA approved, flutemetamol (Vizamyl) and florbetaben (Neuraceq). I use amyloid imaging when I have a symptomatic patient who I think has Alzheimer's disease, and it is really important that I have the right diagnosis. Again, that usually means the patient is young, and I wouldn't want to stop my investigations into the cause of the patient's memory decline unless I was sure it was Alzheimer's. In my VA clinic, we usually do use amyloid imaging when we have a patient younger than 70 years, because Alzheimer's disease is less likely in someone young, as you just heard from Dr. Thor Stein (Chapter 8). Once we have disease-modifying therapies, it may become very important to get these scans in most patients, but we will wait and see what happens with that.

TREATMENT OF ALZHEIMER'S DISEASE DEMENTIA

I wanted to spend a couple of minutes talking about treating these patients. Many of the questions that came up yesterday, particularly from the family members, were about treatments. I want to talk about some of the treatments that have been developed for Alzheimer's disease, and then we will talk about how we can apply these treatments to patients with CTE.

One of the most important points about treatment is that it is critical to get rid of medications that could impair the individual's cognition. Only after removing medications that could harm cognition are we ready to consider medications that could enhance cognition.

There are two FDA-approved classes of medication that can enhance cognition. Cholinesterase inhibitors include donepezil (Aricept and generic), rivastigmine (Exelon and generic), and galantamine (generic). In addition to a traditional pill form, donepezil has an oral dissolving tablet, and rivastigmine has a once-a-day patch. Huperzine A is a cholinesterase inhibitor that is a natural product available at health food stores. There are studies that show it works, although in my experience it's not as potent as our standard drugs. The second class of medications is memantine (Namenda and generic).

Cholinesterase Inhibitors

Cholinesterase inhibitors have been around for a long time, and there is a lot of evidence to show that they

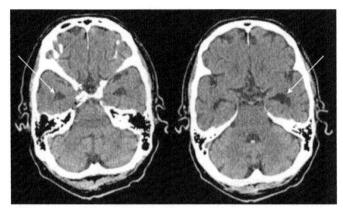

FIG. 9.5 Selected slices of a CT scan of a patient with mild Alzheimer's disease. Note the prominent dilatation of the temporal horns of the lateral ventricles bilaterally (*arrows*). This so-called ex vacuo dilatation (or enlargement due to loss of tissue) of this part of the ventricles is due to the underlying shrinkage of the hippocampi. (From Budson AE, Solomon PR. *Memory Loss, Alzheimer's Disease, and Dementia: A Practical Guide for Clinicians*, 2nd ed. Elsevier; 2016.)

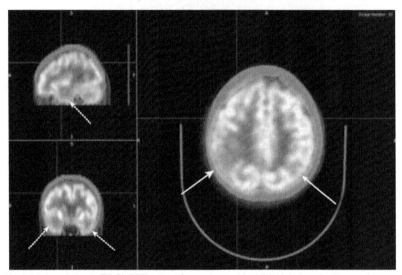

FIG. 9.6 Fluorodeoxyglucose (FDG) PET scan of a patient with mild Alzheimer's disease demonstrating greatly reduced brain metabolism function in right parietal (*thick solid arrow*) and bilateral temporal (*dotted arrows*) regions and more mild reduced metabolism in the left parietal (*thin solid arrow*) region. (From Budson AE, Solomon PR. *Memory Loss, Alzheimer's Disease, and Dementia: A Practical Guide for Clinicians*, 2nd ed. Elsevier; 2016.)

can help improve memory and other aspects of cognition (Fig. 9.8),[5] activities of daily living (Fig. 9.9),[6] and they can even improve behavior[7]—which I think is simply because the patient is a little bit more with it, they know what is going on, they are less likely to get confused or agitated.

In my patients in the clinic I see small but noticeable improvements. A patient with mild Alzheimer's disease dementia might spend less time looking for their keys and glasses. They are going to repeat themselves less often. And they are going to be more able to keep track of what's going on. Because of these types

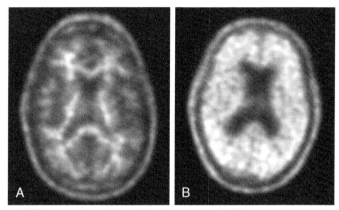

FIG. 9.7 Florbetapir PET scans of an older adult without amyloid (**A**) and a patient with Alzheimer's disease (**B**). Note that in the older adult without amyloid (**A**) the white matter (which takes up the tracer) can be clearly differentiated from the cortex (which does not take up the tracer), but in the patient with Alzheimer's disease (**B**), the white matter and the cortex cannot be differentiated, as both take up the tracer. (From Budson AE, Solomon PR. *Memory Loss, Alzheimer's Disease, and Dementia: A Practical Guide for Clinicians*, 2nd ed. Elsevier; 2016.)

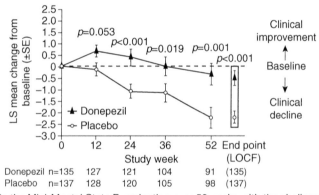

FIG. 9.8 Change in the Mini-Mental State Examination over 52 weeks with the cholinesterase inhibitor donepezil versus placebo. (From Winblad B, Engedal K, Soininen H, et al. A 1-year, randomized, placebo-controlled study of donepezil in patients with mild to moderate AD. *Neurology*. August 14, 2001;57(3):489–495. PMID: 11502918.)

of improvements, they tend to be more engaged and involved in things.

The majority of side effects of the cholinesterase inhibitors are directly related to what happens if you increase the levels of acetylcholine in the body. Most side effects are gastrointestinal, so people can lose their appetite, have nausea, occasional vomiting, and loose stools. Vivid dreams at night are the next most common symptom that patients will tell me about—not nightmares but whatever dreams they have normally can seem very real. Other cholinergic symptoms can include increased salivation, runny nose, muscle cramps, and slowing of the heart. Slowing of the heart rate is important enough that I do get an electrocardiogram on my patients after they are at the highest dose of the cholinesterase inhibitor that I am going to prescribe, to make sure I am not missing any type of heart block.

Goals of Treatment

Now I want to talk about how these drugs work (Fig. 9.10).[1] If we have time here in months to years on the x-axis and function on the y-axis (which can be memory function, global function, or whatever treatment

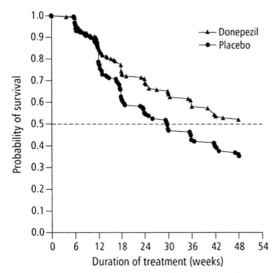

FIG. 9.9 Time to clinically evident functional decline over 52 weeks with the cholinesterase inhibitor donepezil versus placebo. (From Mohs RC, Doody RS, Morris JC, et al. A 1-year, placebo-controlled preservation of function survival study of donepezil in AD patients. *Neurology.* August 14, 2001;57(3):481–488. Erratum in: Neurology. November 27, 2001;57(10):1942. PMID: 11502917.)

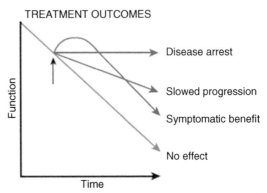

FIG. 9.10 Outcomes for different types of treatments in neurodegenerative diseases, including those that can arrest the disease, slow progression, or provide a symptomatic benefit. (From Budson AE, Solomon PR. *Memory Loss, Alzheimer's Disease, and Dementia: A Practical Guide for Clinicians,* 2nd ed. Elsevier; 2016.)

outcome you want), if we start with an untreated patient they are going to decline at a certain theoretical slope. When we intervene with a treatment, what we would love to do would be to completely arrest the disease, to stop it in its tracks. Unfortunately, we don't have anything that can do that, and nor do I see anything on the horizon than can stop Alzheimer's or any other neurodegenerative disease. Well, if we cannot arrest the disease maybe we can slow it down. There are a lot of compounds that are in clinical trials right now for Alzheimer's that may be able to do that, but they have not been proven to do so quite yet. What we have currently are medications that produce a symptomatic benefit, including both the cholinesterase inhibitors and memantine.

A symptomatic benefit means that the patient will show an actual improvement but then a decline along a similar slope as if they were untreated. Note, however, that they are always better off being up on the symptomatic treatment curve than down on the no effect curve, even though the slopes of decline are the same. It is very important that both patients and families understand this point. What will generally happen if they don't understand is that initially they

will see the benefit—the improvement—and the family comes in and says, "Thank you so much, Dr. Budson, my mother is so much better! I am so glad we came to see you and started her on this medicine." This is a great result, but then maybe a year and a half later the patient's cognition has declined past where they were when they first came to see me and there is a whole other attitude that emerges: "What is going on, Dr. Budson? Now my mother is getting worse! I want a different medication! I want another MRI scan!" Patients and families need to understand that just because an individual is getting worse doesn't mean that the medication isn't working.

Turning the Clock Back on Memory Loss

So, here is the way I talk with families about what these symptomatic medications do. I talk about "turning back the clock" on memory problems. What the studies show is that approximately 25% to 30% of patients show an improvement that is equivalent to turning back the clock on memory problems by approximately 1 year. About 50% to 60% of patients show an improvement equivalent to turning back the clock on memory problems about 6 months, and the remainder show either no improvement or just a very small improvement.

I give everybody a trial of cholinesterase inhibitors and I try to figure out if they're working in my individual patient. How do I know if the medication is working? In patients who are only mildly impaired

I can ask them how they think they are doing. Asking family members is usually the most important metric both because they are often good observers and because we want to see if the medication improves the patients' daily life, not just paper and pencil testing. But with that said, I do recommend testing the patient before and after the medication using the Montreal Cognitive Assessment or a Mini-Mental State Examination or whatever cognitive measure you like to do.

Here are a couple figures with actual data from cholinesterase inhibitors. In Fig. 9.8 you can see the control group showing a fairly straight line of decline. The donepezil group shows a bump up and then a decline along a similar slope. You can see that the average patient in this study had the clock turned back by 36 weeks—because that is where the donepezil group crossed baseline—but some patients showed a full 52 weeks of "turning back of the clock" as you can see from the error bar crossing the baseline at 52 weeks in the donepezil group.[5] Fig. 9.9 shows that function is improved and, of course, that is what we are really trying to accomplish—if function is improved then everyone is happy.[6]

Continue Cholinesterase Inhibitors as Long as There Is Function to Preserve

Now the question frequently comes up, how long should we use cholinesterase inhibitors? Should we stop when the patient reaches the moderate to severe stage of dementia, whether the dementia is due to Alzheimer's or CTE? Howard and colleagues did the following study to answer this question, at least in Alzheimer's.[8] In a randomized, double-blind, placebo-controlled fashion they took patients who were on donepezil 10 mg and they either replaced their donepezil with placebo or kept them on it, and they either added memantine or they didn't. Those individuals who stayed on active donepezil did better than those who had the placebo donepezil, and those patients who had memantine added actually did the best of all. Note, however, that, although the memantine group didn't end up being statistically significant, the donepezil group did. In fact, the authors concluded that, "In patients with moderate or severe Alzheimer's disease, continued treatment with donepezil was associated with cognitive benefits that exceeded the minimum clinically important difference and with significant functional benefits over the course of 12 months." So, not only was there a statistically significant effect, the magnitude of the effect met their clinically significant effect threshold as well. So, the result of this study was that the cholinesterase inhibitor made a difference in patients' lives. My recommendation is to continue cholinesterase inhibitors in patients as long as there is quality of life to preserve.

Memantine for Moderate to Severe Dementia

Let's talk for a minute or two about memantine. Memantine is approved for use in patients with moderate to severe Alzheimer's disease dementia either with or without cholinesterase inhibitors, although I definitely recommend using it with cholinesterase inhibitors. It is known to be an uncompetitive N-methyl-D-aspartate (NMDA) receptor antagonist that modulates glutamate receptors, but it also enhances dopamine activity. My own suspicion is it's the dopamine activity enhancement that produces its main pharmacological effect in humans in the doses that we give it. Whatever the mechanism, studies have shown that in patients with moderate to severe Alzheimer's disease there is improvement or less decline in cognition, activities of daily living, and behavior—especially if you combine it with cholinesterase inhibitors like donepezil.

I want to mention to all you prescribers out there, memantine does not seem to improve memory, with data coming both from the studies as well as my experience. It does improve other aspects of cognition: patients are more alert, talkative, engaged, and outgoing. They tend to be "brighter." All these things are ones that patients with moderate to severe dementia need help with. There are relatively few side effects of memantine. In the published studies, none were actually more frequent than those observed with placebo. Side effects that I and others have observed, however, include drowsiness and confusion. Drowsiness and confusion are tricky side effects because *all* my patients with moderate to severe dementia have some sort of confusion. Because of this fact, for me to continue the medication I want to hear the families say that the memantine has really made a difference, it really produced improvement. If, on the other hand, they say, "maybe he is a bit better but I am not sure," then I generally stop it. You really want to hear that the patient has had a positive benefit to continue with it. Otherwise I would recommend getting rid of it—the last thing we want to do is to cause drowsiness and confusion in one of our patients with dementia!

MILD COGNITIVE IMPAIRMENT

Let's take a look at another patient. This individual is a 72-year-old man with mild memory complaints. He was the CEO of a large company, a very bright and successful guy. He found that, although he was previously able to remember his schedule in his head, now his secretary needed to remind him about his appointments or he would miss them. He also found that instead of being able to remember the content of meetings in his head, he now needed to take a lot more notes. He became gradually and slowly worse over 2 years. However, he never forgot anything critically important. He didn't have word-finding problems or other cognitive difficulties. He did have isolated problems with memory on formal testing. This patient has mild cognitive impairment, more commonly referred to as an MCI.

Diagnostic Criteria for Mild Cognitive Impairment

Box 9.3 shows the National Institute on Aging—Alzheimer's Association criteria for MCI due to any disorder, as well as MCI due to Alzheimer's disease. For MCI, there must be a change in cognition noticed by the patient, the informant (usually a family member), or you as the clinician. There needs to be cognitive testing showing impairment in one or more cognitive domains, typically memory. But the patient must have preservation of independence, in other words, they cannot be demented.

OK, so once we know from these general criteria that the patient has MCI, how do we know if it's due to Alzheimer's disease? We first want to rule out other causes of MCI. Next we want to see a slow, gradual, insidious decline. Lastly, we want to see if there are any genetic risk factors that may predispose the patient to Alzheimer's disease. The DSM-5 criteria for mild neurocognitive disorder, in general, and for mild neurocognitive disorder due to Alzheimer's disease, in particular, are very similar to the National Institute on Aging—Alzheimer's Association criteria.

Prognosis of Mild Cognitive Impairment

Now what we find in MCI is that the studies show that between approximately 50% and 70% of patients with a diagnosis of MCI will progress to dementia, either Alzheimer's disease or another disorder, at a rate of about 15% per year. Note that these numbers also mean that the other 30% to 50% stay stable or actually improve. Maybe they had depression. Maybe they had medication side effects.

BOX 9.3

National Institute on Aging—Alzheimer's Association Clinical and Cognitive Criteria for MCI due to AD

ESTABLISH CLINICAL AND COGNITIVE CRITERIA FOR MCI

- Cognitive concern reflecting a change in cognition reported by the patient or informant or clinician (i.e., historical or observed evidence of decline over time)
- Objective evidence of impairment in one or more cognitive domains, typically including memory (i.e., formal or bedside testing to establish level of cognitive function in multiple domains)
- Preservation of independence in functional abilities
- Not demented

EXAMINE ETIOLOGY OF MCI CONSISTENT WITH AD PATHOPHYSIOLOGICAL PROCESS

- Rule out vascular, traumatic, medical causes of cognitive decline, where possible.
- Provide evidence of longitudinal decline in cognition, when feasible.
- Report history consistent with AD genetic factors, where relevant.

AD, Alzheimer's disease; *MCI*, mild cognitive impairment.
Adapted from Albert MS, DeKosky ST, Dickson D, et al. The diagnosis of mild cognitive impairment due to Alzheimer's disease: recommendations from the National Institute on Aging-Alzheimer's Association workgroups on diagnostic guidelines for Alzheimer's disease. *Alzheimer's and Dementia*. 2011;7:270–279.

Treatment of Mild Cognitive Impairment

There are no FDA-approved medications for the treatment of MCI, but I do recommend trying a cholinesterase inhibitor if memory is the major problem and the patient is interested in trying it. Petersen and colleagues conducted a study that demonstrates that Alzheimer's disease dementia can be delayed by at least 1 year using donepezil 10 mg daily.[9]

DEMENTIA WITH LEWY BODIES

Let's look at another patient. Here is someone who is a bit younger, a 65-year-old man. He came in to see me for memory problems, but he also had signs of Parkinson's. He had masked facies and a shuffling gait. He had cogwheeling, which means when I checked his tone in his arm it was not only stiff but it was also ratchety. He also had very prominent visual hallucinations of people and of animals, and at the time I first

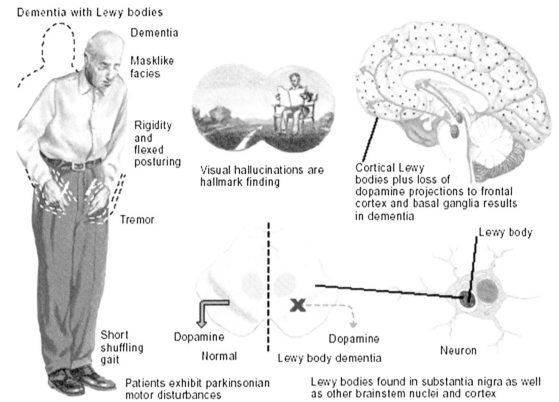

FIG. 9.11 Major clinical and pathological abnormalities in dementia with Lewy bodies. (Netter illustration from www.netterimages.com. Copyright Elsevier Inc. All rights reserved.)

saw him, he saw them fairly regularly—at least once a day—although he didn't tell anyone about them. He knew that the images weren't real, and he was afraid that people would think he was crazy if he told anyone. So, it's very important to ask the patient if they are experiencing hallucinations. He also had visual perception defects. He had difficulty, for example, telling apart different types of money—he couldn't distinguish a one-dollar bill from a ten-dollar bill. His wife also noted that he would wake her up at night kicking and moving around in his sleep.

I'm sure you've all figured out the diagnosis by now. This is a classic case of dementia with Lewy bodies or Parkinson's disease dementia. The main difference between these two disorders is that in Parkinson's disease dementia, the Parkinson's disease starts first, by at least a year, and the other cognitive and behavioral symptoms begin later. In dementia with Lewy bodies, either the two types of symptoms

start at roughly at the same time or sometimes the cognitive and behavioral symptoms (including hallucinations) start first and then the Parkinson's signs and symptoms come later. Fig. 9.11 shows you some of the major features of the disorder, and Box 9.4 shows the full criteria for diagnosis.[10]

Pathologically, the way I think about it is that in Parkinson's disease there are Lewy bodies in the substantia nigra of the midbrain, depleting dopamine and thus producing parkinsonism, but, in addition, in dementia with Lewy bodies there are Lewy bodies throughout the cortex. We believe that it is the cortical Lewy bodies in the occipital lobes causing visual perception dysfunction plus a sleep cycle disturbance that produces the prominent visual hallucinations—they may be dream phenomena breaking into waking consciousness. The sleep cycle disturbance is certainly present, because the reason why he was kicking his wife and moving around in bed is that he had rapid eye movement (REM) sleep

---

BOX 9.4
Selected Revised Criteria for Clinical Diagnosis of Dementia With Lewy Bodies

1. Essential for a diagnosis:
   a. Dementia defined as progressive cognitive decline sufficient to interfere with normal social or occupational function. Impairment in attention, executive function, and visuospatial ability are often prominent. Memory impairment may or may not be prominent initially.
2. Core features (two are sufficient for a diagnosis of probable dementia with Lewy bodies; one is sufficient for a possible diagnosis):
   a. Fluctuating cognition (pronounced variations in attention and alertness)
   b. Visual hallucinations (recurrent, well-formed, detailed, of people and/or animals, often initially present around transitions between sleep and wake)
   c. Spontaneous features of parkinsonism
3. Suggestive features (one or more plus one core feature allows a probable diagnosis; one or more without any core features allows a possible diagnosis):
   a. Rapid eye movement sleep behavior disorder

   b. Severe neuroleptic sensitivity
   c. Low dopamine transporter uptake in basal ganglia demonstrated by SPECT or PET imaging
4. Supportive features (commonly present but have not been proven to have diagnostic specificity):
   a. Repeated falls
   b. Transient unexplained loss of consciousness
   c. Orthostatic hypotension
   d. Reduced occipital activity and generalized low uptake on SPECT/PET perfusion scan
5. A diagnosis of dementia with Lewy bodies is less likely:
   a. In the presence of clinically significant cerebrovascular disease noted on examination or radiology study
   b. If parkinsonism appears only for the first time at a stage of severe dementia
   c. In the presence of any other disorder sufficient to account for some or all of the clinical picture

Adapted from McKeith IG, Dickson DW, Lowe J, et al. Diagnosis and management of dementia with Lewy bodies: third report of the DLB Consortium. *Neurology*. 2005;65:1863–1872.

---

behavior disorder—he was not paralyzed during REM sleep, which most of us are when we are dreaming.

In a straightforward case like this one, no further workup is needed; the diagnosis is very clear. If you are not sure, however, an FDG PET or ^{99m}Tc-hexamethylpropyleneamine oxime (HMPAO) single-photon emission computed tomography (SPECT) scan can be helpful. Fig. 9.12 shows the characteristic occipital hypofunction that is typically seen.

Regarding treatment, the cholinesterase inhibitor rivastigmine is actually FDA approved for Parkinson's disease dementia, and in my experience any of the cholinesterase inhibitors can be helpful,[11] as can memantine.

VASCULAR DEMENTIA

The next patient is a 74-year-old man with a 6-year history of "small TIAs." When I asked the family, "What do you mean he has 'small TIAs'?," they told me that in a single day he may have a sudden decline in his speech, his handwriting, and his walking, which would get better, but not all the way back to baseline. I scratched my head and said to myself, "Well, if it's

not getting all the way back to baseline, then it's not a '*transient* ischemic attack,'" which is what TIA stands for. So maybe the episodes were more than TIAs. The family also noted that he had memory problems. They would ask him to do things and he would forget. He would sometimes show up for appointments and family gatherings on the wrong day or in the wrong place. Interestingly, he remembered the last Red Sox game really well, which told me that his memory was quite variable. He did have a lot of trouble recalling specific details, but he was generally oriented to time and place and what was going on. He also had poor walking and early incontinence.

There is certainly a large differential diagnosis that could be causing these symptoms, but it turned out that he had a vascular dementia. The clue was that he was having what the family called TIAs, which were actually small strokes. Box 9.5 shows the full diagnostic criteria for vascular dementia.[12] Fig. 9.13 shows his MRI scan showing small strokes throughout the deep gray structures, including the thalamus and basal ganglia. You can also see how the frontal subcortical white matter tracts are just devastated by small vessel ischemic disease.

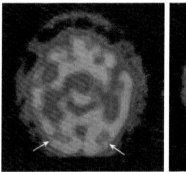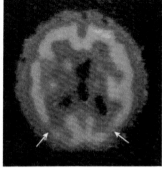

FIG. 9.12 Single-photon emission computed tomography scan in a patient with dementia with Lewy bodies. Note the decreased occipital function (*arrows*). (From Budson AE, Solomon PR. *Memory Loss, Alzheimer's Disease, and Dementia: A Practical Guide for Clinicians*, 2nd ed. Elsevier; 2016.)

BOX 9.5
International Society for Vascular Behavioral and Cognitive Disorders Criteria for Vascular Cognitive Disorders

CRITERIA FOR MILD COGNITIVE DISORDER AND DEMENTIA (OR MAJOR COGNITIVE DISORDER)

Mild Cognitive Disorder

1. Acquired decline from a documented or inferred previous level of performance in ≥1 cognitive domains (attention and processing speed, frontal/executive function, learning and memory, language, visuoconstructional-perceptual ability, praxis-gnosis-body schema, social cognition) as evidenced by the following:

   a. Concerns of a patient, knowledgeable informant, or a clinician of mild levels of decline from a previous level of cognitive functioning and

   b. Evidence of modest deficits (1 to 2 standard deviations below norms) on objective cognitive assessment based on a validated measure of neurocognitive function in ≥1 cognitive domains.

2. The cognitive deficits are not sufficient to interfere with independence in instrumental activities of daily living, but greater effort, compensatory strategies, or accommodation may be required.

Dementia or Major Cognitive Disorder

1. Evidence of substantial cognitive decline from a documented or inferred previous level of performance in ≥1 cognitive domains based on:

   a. Concerns of the patient, a knowledgeable informant, or the clinician of significant decline in specific abilities; and

   b. Clear and significant deficits (≥2 standard deviations below the mean) in objective assessment based on a validated objective measure of neurocognitive function in ≥1 cognitive domains.

2. The cognitive deficits are sufficient to interfere with independence in instrumental activities of daily living.

EVIDENCE FOR PREDOMINANTLY VASCULAR ETIOLOGY OF COGNITIVE IMPAIRMENT

1. One of the following clinical features:

   a. The onset of the cognitive deficits is temporally related to ≥1 cerebrovascular events, as evidenced by one of the following:

      i. Documented history of a stroke, with cognitive decline temporally associated with the event

      ii. Physical signs consistent with stroke

   b. Evidence for decline is prominent in speed of information processing, complex attention, and/or frontal/executive functioning in the absence of history of a stroke or transient ischemic attack. One of the following features is additionally present:

      i. Early presence of a gait disturbance (small-step gait or *marche à petits pas*, or magnetic, apraxic-ataxic, or parkinsonian gait); this may also manifest as unsteadiness and frequent, unprovoked falls

      ii. Early urinary frequency, urgency, and other urinary symptoms not explained by urologic disease

      iii. Personality and mood changes: abulia, depression, or emotional incontinence

2. Presence of significant neuroimaging (MRI or CT) evidence of cerebrovascular disease (one of the following):

   a. One large vessel infarct is sufficient for Mild Vascular Cognitive Disorder, and ≥2 large vessel infarcts are generally necessary for Vascular Dementia (or Major Vascular Cognitive Disorder)

Continued

b. An extensive or strategically placed single infarct, typically in the thalamus or basal ganglia, may be sufficient for Vascular Dementia (or Major Vascular Cognitive Disorder)

c. Multiple lacunar infarcts (>2) outside the brainstem; 1 to 2 lacunes may be sufficient if strategically placed or in combination with extensive white matter lesions

d. Extensive and confluent white matter lesions

e. Strategically placed intracerebral hemorrhage or ≥2 intracerebral hemorrhages

f. Combination of the above

EXCLUSION CRITERIA (FOR MILD AND MAJOR VASCULAR COGNITIVE DISORDER)

1. History
   a. Early onset of memory deficit and progressive worsening of memory and other cognitive functions, such as language, motor skills, and perception, in the absence of corresponding focal lesions on brain imaging or history of vascular events

b. Early and prominent parkinsonian features suggestive of Lewy body disease

c. History strongly suggestive of another primary neurological disorder sufficient to explain the cognitive impairment

2. Neuroimaging
   a. Absent or minimal cerebrovascular lesions on CT or MRI

3. Other medical disorders severe enough to account for memory and related symptoms:
   a. Other disease of sufficient severity to cause cognitive impairment
   b. Major depression, with a temporal association between cognitive impairment and the likely onset of depression
   c. Toxic and metabolic abnormalities, all of which may require specific investigations

Adapted from Sachdev P, Kalaria R, O'Brien J, et al. Diagnostic criteria for vascular cognitive disorders: a VASCOG statement. *Alzheimer Disease and Associated Disorders*. 2014;28:206–218.

Cholinesterase inhibitors are not FDA approved for vascular dementia, but there are studies that show they are helpful, so we often prescribe them.[13] Sometimes memantine can be helpful as well, and it is actually approved for vascular dementia in Europe.[14]

NORMAL-PRESSURE HYDROCEPHALUS

This next patient was a 76-year-old woman who presented with poor cognition over 6 to 12 months. She had very impaired attention—it was difficult for her to focus on a conversation. I tested her myself in the clinic, and she was having difficulty focusing on the testing. She was also incontinent of urine, and she had a magnetic gate disorder—when I asked her what was wrong with her walking she actually told me that her feet felt like they were stuck to the floor. This walking is also called a frontal gait disorder, and the French call it a *marche à petits pas*, meaning "walk of little steps." She had very poor free recall of information, but if you tested her with recognition she did pretty well.

This patient had normal-pressure hydrocephalus. See Box 9.6 for the full diagnostic criteria.[15] Fig. 9.14 shows her CT scan with very large, balloon-like ventricles, and the hypodensity you can see around the ventricles

is actually trans-ependymal flow of CSF or spinal fluid that is pushing its way out into the tissue. To confirm the diagnosis and also get a sense as to whether the patient would respond to treatment, we typically do daily large-volume lumbar punctures over 3 days looking for a quantitative improvement in walking speed. (See Chapter 10 for additional detail on lumbar punctures.)

The treatment is a ventriculoperitoneal shunt. The studies suggest that, with shunting, the gait disorder and the incontinence improve and the cognition will stay stable, so it is important to identify and treat these patients as early as possible. One can also consider symptomatic therapies for any residual cognitive symptoms.

FRONTOTEMPORAL DEMENTIA

The next patient was a 78-year-old man with memory and behavior problems. For 3 to 4 years he had difficulty remembering information and became easily confused. About a year before I saw him he began exhibiting behaviors that were uncharacteristic of him: he was watching pornography in the living room and not caring if other people were observing him. He was telling sexually explicit jokes in front of his family in an inappropriate way. He was depressed and apathetic.

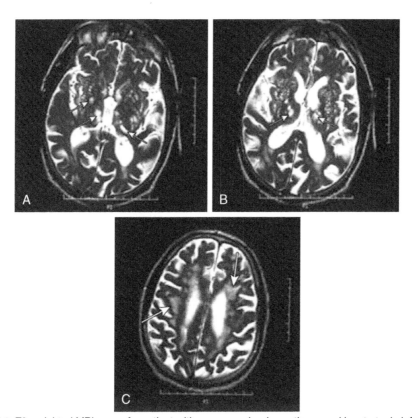

FIG. 9.13 T2-weighted MRI scan of a patient with pure vascular dementia caused by strategic infarcts and small vessel ischemic disease. Note the multiple bright areas in the deep gray structures of the brain, including basal ganglia and thalamus (**A** and **B**), and the periventricular subcortical white matter (**C**), indicating strategic infarcts (*thin arrows*, not all infarcts indicated) and small vessel ischemic disease (*thick arrows*, not all disease indicated). (From Budson AE, Solomon PR. *Memory Loss, Alzheimer's Disease, and Dementia: A Practical Guide for Clinicians*, 2nd ed. Elsevier; 2016.)

He would often pace around the room with nervous energy. He easily lost control of his temper.

This is a patient with a frontotemporal dementia. It is a particularly important disorder to mention here because it can be easily confused with CTE. In fact, many patients with CTE would actually meet the formal criteria for frontotemporal dementia (Box 9.7). Fig. 9.15 shows his ^{99m}Tc-HMPAO SPECT scan, which is one of the ways we knew we had the right diagnosis. Note the relatively smooth confluent area of hypofunction in the frontal lobe.

TREATING FRONTAL LOBE SYMPTOMS

Now I want to switch gears here a little bit and talk about how we treat frontal lobe symptoms in any disorder, including frontotemporal dementia, vascular dementia, Alzheimer's disease, and, of course, CTE.

Pseudobulbar Affect

The first symptom I would like to discuss is called pseudobulbar affect. I am quite sure that several of the CTE patients we saw in the videos yesterday had this symptom. It is when emotional expressions—usually crying or laughing—occur with either minimal provocation or for no reason at all. So, the individual may spontaneously laugh or cry, and other times it may be that the topic is sad but if the individual didn't have their neurodegenerative disease they would not have broken down into tears when they were talking about it. Pseudobulbar affect is very common in many forms of dementias, including Alzheimer's disease and vascular dementia. I think it is quite common in CTE as well.

Pseudobulbar affect can sometimes be difficult to identify. You have to probe for it. I confess that, although I was familiar with it, before this new medication to treat it came along, I didn't always ask the right questions to

---

BOX 9.6
Criteria for Probable Normal-Pressure Hydrocephalus

1. History must include:
   a. Insidious onset
   b. Age 40 years or older
   c. Duration of symptoms greater than 3 months
   d. No evidence of an antecedent event known to cause hydrocephalus
   e. Progression of symptoms over time
   f. No other neurological, psychiatric, or medical condition that can explain the presenting signs and symptoms
2. Brain imaging (CT or MRI) must show
   a. Ventricular enlargement not solely caused by atrophy or congenital enlargement
   b. No visible obstruction of cerebrospinal fluid flow
   c. Callosal angle of 40 degrees or greater (rounding of the ventricular contours)
   d. Evidence of periventricular trans-ependymal flow of cerebrospinal fluid
   e. Aqueductal or fourth ventricular flow void on MRI
3. Supportive brain imaging (CT or MRI) findings include
   a. Prior brain imaging study showing smaller ventricular size
   b. Radionuclide cisternogram showing delayed clearance of radiotracer
   c. Cine MRI showing increased ventricular flow
   d. SPECT-acetazolamide challenge showing decreased perfusion not altered by acetazolamide
4. Clinical findings of gait/balance disturbance plus either cognitive impairment or urinary symptoms or both:
   a. Gait disturbance that includes at least two of the following (not entirely attributable to other conditions):
      i. Decreased step height
      ii. Decreased step length
      iii. Decreased cadence (speed of walking)
      iv. Increased trunk sway during walking
      v. Widened standing base
      vi. Toes turned outward on walking
      vii. Spontaneous or provoked retropulsion
      viii. En bloc turning (needing 3+ steps for turning 180 degrees)
      ix. Impaired walking balance, tested by 2+ corrections needed for tandem gait of eight steps
   b. Cognitive impairment that includes at least two of the following (not entirely attributable to other conditions):
      i. Psychomotor slowing (increased latency of response)
      ii. Decreased fine motor speed
      iii. Decreased fine motor accuracy
      iv. Difficulty dividing or maintaining attention
      v. Impaired memory recall, especially for recent events
      vi. Executive dysfunction, including impairment in multistep procedures, working memory, abstractions, similarities, and insight
      vii. Behavioral or personality changes
   c. Urinary incontinence not entirely attributable to other conditions consisting of either
      i. Episodic urinary incontinence
      ii. Persistent urinary incontinence
      iii. Urinary and fecal incontinence
      Or any two of the following:
      iv. Frequent perception of the need to void
      v. Urinary frequency
      vi. Nocturia greater than two times per night
5. Physiological
   a. CSF opening pressure of 70 to 245 mm H_2O (5 to 18 mm Hg)

Adapted from Relkin N, Marmarou A, Klinge P, et al. Diagnosing idiopathic normal-pressure hydrocephalus. *Neurosurgery*. 2005;57:S4–S16.

---

see if it was present. The typical scenario is that a patient would come to my office and the family would say, "I think my mother is really depressed; she has been crying a lot." So, I used to say, "OK, maybe there is some depression present, I'll prescribe your mother an antidepressant medication," usually a selective serotonin reuptake inhibitor (SSRI), and send them on their way. Now I have gotten smarter. Now I turn to the patient and I ask, "Mrs. Jones, your family notes that you are crying more. Are you feeling sad?" And sometimes just asking this question would be enough for Mrs. Jones to start crying. But about half of the time Mrs. Jones responds, "No, I am not feeling sad, and I don't know why I am crying." That's pseudobulbar affect, and it is something that we clinicians need to ask about, just like we do with many other signs and symptoms.

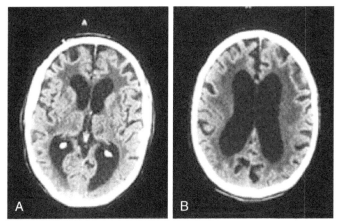

FIG. 9.14 CT scan from a patient with normal-pressure hydrocephalus. In this example, there is some cortical atrophy, but note the overly large, "ballooned-out" expansion of the ventricular system in both slices. Note also the trans-ependymal cerebrospinal fluid that appears hypodense anterior to the frontal horns of the lateral ventricles (**A**) and surrounding the ventricles (**B**). This patient improved dramatically after a diagnostic lumbar puncture and subsequently received a ventricular-peritoneal shunt. (From Budson AE, Solomon PR. *Memory Loss, Alzheimer's Disease, and Dementia: A Practical Guide for Clinicians*, 2nd ed. Elsevier; 2016.)

The reason it is important to figure out whether it is depression or pseudobulbar affect is that the treatments are different. There is a relatively new FDA-approved medication to treat pseudobulbar affect that is present in any disorder. So, it actually doesn't matter what the underlying neurologic diagnosis is as long as the patient has the symptom of pseudobulbar affect. The treatment is a combination pill of 20 mg of dextromethorphan and 10 mg of quinidine; the brand name is Nuedexta. The way it works is that the dextromethorphan is the active ingredient and the quinidine stops the metabolism of dextromethorphan so it stays in the bloodstream and the brain longer. People generally tolerate it just fine; the only serious side effects are from the quinidine, which is an antiarrhythmic. I should note, however, that the quinidine dose used is much lower than the dose used as an antiarrhythmic.

Agitation

Let's talk about managing agitation. This symptom is also one that comes up very frequently in CTE. Our families yesterday talked about problems with agitation. We also saw agitation happening on the videos that Dr. McKee and others showed us of individuals with CTE.

So, the first thing I always try to do is to understand the underlying cause of the agitation—there is probably nothing more important regarding its treatment than to first figure out why it is happening. Once you

understand why it is happening then you can initiate the right treatment. I also always start with nonpharmacological therapies. We use the three R's—Reassure, Reconsider, and Redirect. So, the caregiver needs to *reassure* the patient that everything is OK. *Reconsider* means consider things from the patients' point of view. *Redirect* means that instead of telling the patient, "You can't leave the house and go home because you already are home," you need to get them distracted by something else: show them something on TV show, show them a picture book or a photo album. Get them talking about the old days or engaged in a hobby, anything at all.

If the agitation is due to anxiety—which it often is—an SSRI with anxiolytic properties, can be helpful. I typically use either serotonin or escitalopram. Those SSRIs tend to work well, and there are actually studies showing that both can be beneficial in individuals with dementia. Escitalopram has the strongest data, although I've had the best personal experience prescribing sertraline.

Sleep cycle disturbances are very common. Families frequently say to me, "Dad is agitated at night—he is up at 4 a.m. wandering around the house, getting dressed, making noise, I can't get any sleep!" I will respond, "Well, tell me about his day, and when he goes to sleep." They will say, "We put him to bed around 8 p.m." So, then I will have to explain to them that if you put him to bed at 8 p.m., by 4 a.m. he has had

---

BOX 9.7
International Behavioral Variant Frontotemporal Dementia Criteria

1. Shows progressive deterioration of behavior and/or cognition by observation or history (as provided by knowledgeable informant)
2. *Possible behavioral variant frontotemporal dementia*: Three of the following behavioral/cognitive symptoms (a to f) must be present as persistent or recurrent events:
   a. Early[a] behavioral disinhibition (one of the following must be present):
      i. Socially inappropriate behavior
      ii. Loss of manners or decorum
      iii. Impulsive, rash, or careless actions
   b. Early apathy or inertia (one of the following must be present):
      i. Apathy: loss of interest, drive, or motivation
      ii. Inertia: decreased initiation of behavior
   c. Early loss of sympathy or empathy (one of the following must be present):
      i. Diminished response to other people's needs or feelings: positive rating should be based on specific examples that reflect a lack of understanding or indifference to other people's feelings
      ii. Diminished social interest, interrelatedness, or personal warmth: general decrease in social engagement
   d. Early perseverative, stereotyped, or compulsive/ritualistic behavior (one of the following must be present):
      i. Simple repetitive movements
      ii. Complex, compulsive, or ritualistic behaviors
      iii. Stereotypy of speech
   e. Hyperorality and dietary changes (one of the following must be present):
      i. Altered food preferences
      ii. Binge eating, increased consumption of alcohol or cigarettes
      iii. Oral exploration or consumption of inedible objects
   f. Neuropsychological profile: executive/generation deficits with relative sparing of memory and visuospatial functions (all of the following must be present):
      i. Deficits in executive tasks
      ii. Relative sparing of episodic memory (compared with degree of executive dysfunction)
      iii. Relative sparing of visuospatial skills (compared with degree of executive dysfunction)
3. *Probable behavioral variant frontotemporal dementia*: All criteria must be met
   a. Meets criteria for possible behavioral variant frontotemporal dementia
   b. Exhibits significant functional decline (by caregiver report, clinician rating, or functional questionnaire)
   c. Imaging results consistent with behavioral variant frontotemporal dementia
      i. Frontal and/or anterior temporal atrophy on CT or MRI and/or
      ii. Frontal and/or anterior temporal hypoperfusion or hypometabolism on SPECT or PET
4. Behavioral variant frontotemporal dementia with definite frontotemporal lobar degeneration pathology. Criterion a and either b or c must be present:
   a. Meets criteria for possible or probable behavioral variant frontotemporal dementia
   b. Histopathological evidence of frontotemporal lobar degeneration on biopsy or at postmortem
   c. Presence of a known pathogenic mutation
5. Exclusionary criteria for behavioral variant frontotemporal dementia. Criteria a and b must be answered negatively. Criteria c can be positive for possible (but not probable) behavioral variant frontotemporal dementia.
   a. Pattern of deficits is better accounted for by other nondegenerative nervous system or medical disorders
   b. Behavioral disturbance is better accounted for by a psychiatric diagnosis
   c. Biomarkers strongly indicative of Alzheimer's disease or other neurodegenerative process

[a] Early refers to symptoms within the first 3 years.
Adapted from Rascovsky K, Hodges JR, Knopman D, et al. Sensitivity of revised diagnostic criteria for the behavioral variant of frontotemporal dementia. *Brain*. 2011;134:2456–2477 and LaMarre AK, Rascovsky K, Bostrom A, et al. Interrater reliability of the new criteria for behavioral variant frontotemporal dementia. *Neurology*. 2013;80:1973–1977.

---

8 h of sleep, so it is not surprising that he is awake—he probably just had enough sleep! Then they complain, "How am I going to have time for myself if I don't put him to bed at 8 p.m.?" So, I explain to the family, "You can make the decision regarding when you want him to sleep, but I am not going to give him a medication to put him to sleep for 12 h when he only needs 8 h and is already getting enough sleep at night." If the problem is that the patient is falling asleep during the day, I will sometimes use a small dose of a stimulant like Ritalin

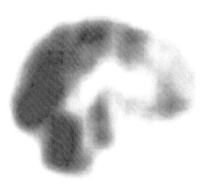

FIG. 9.15 Midsagittal slice of a single-photon emission computed tomography scan in a patient with behavioral frontotemporal dementia. Note the reduced activity in the front of the brain (right side of image) relative to more posterior regions. (From Budson AE, Solomon PR. *Memory Loss, Alzheimer's Disease, and Dementia: A Practical Guide for Clinicians*, 2nd ed. Elsevier; 2016.)

or Provigil to help keep them awake during the day—they will even be more alert—and then they can fall asleep at night at a normal time. A short nap for about 30 min—never more than 60—is also fine. Exercise during the day—even just walking for 30 min—will also help them sleep well through the night.

If you have tried all these things and more and there is still a problem with agitation during the day, a low dose of risperidone is sometimes helpful. For nighttime agitation, I've been using the side effects of medication to help patients go to sleep. I might use a very small dose of trazodone or quetiapine—but again, I really try to stay away from any sedating medications if I can.

Recently there is evidence the combination of dextromethorphan and quinidine (Nuedexta) that I described as treatment for pseudobulbar affect can also be beneficial for agitation. This was a study published in the *Journal of the American Medical Association* just last year showing that patients showed fewer neuropsychiatric symptoms with Nuedexta compared to placebo.[16]

CHRONIC TRAUMATIC ENCEPHALOPATHY

Let's take a look at one more patient. This is a patient in my clinic that I have now followed for about 4 years. She is a 59-year-old woman with forgetfulness. Unfortunately, she had a long history of domestic abuse that was described to me as frequent blows to the head and occasional concussions that started in her early 20s. When I first met her she was described as very tearful, but she also had emotional blunting—she didn't show full emotion through her face. She had a lot of language

deficits, including word-finding difficulties and frequent paraphasic errors, including phonemic and neologistic errors. She also had a lot of trouble in daily life. She would put plastic Tupperware into the oven. She would try to cook with the wrong ingredients.

On exam she had signs of Parkinson's disease, including increased tone, bilateral resting tremor, cogwheeling, and Myerson's sign—when I tapped on her forehead she kept blinking; the normal response is you blink initially and then you stop. She also had very brisk reflexes. Over the 4 years that I followed her, she became progressively more aphasic and more apraxic—she couldn't perform skilled motor movements properly. She also showed more signs of frontal lobe dysfunction over the years.

Structural Imaging in CTE

Fig. 9.16 shows her MRI scan, and I want to point out a couple of different features. First, there is atrophy of the anterior temporal lobes, which is asymmetric, left much more than right, and there is medial temporal lobe atrophy as well—hippocampal and temporal lobe atrophy leading to ex vacuo expansion of the temporal horn of the lateral ventricles (Fig. 9.16A and B). Note that her occipital lobes are perfect, so we are getting a hint that there is multifocal atrophy—it is not global atrophy. In Fig. 9.16C, we see asymmetric left-sided atrophy in the frontal lobe, the same side of the head as the temporal lobe atrophy. Note that the other parts of the cortex you can see on this image are looking relatively fine. But here we see she has a cavum septum pellucidum and also cavum vergae, which is the bottom part of the cavum. Fig. 9.16D shows another slice with this very large cavum of the septum, and in Fig. 9.16E you can see the fenestrations—the holes in the septum—you lose the nice line of the septum on this slice. Fig. 9.16F is another slice to show you the cavum and left greater than right cortical atrophy, and Fig. 9.16G shows focal left frontal atrophy. So, in summary, we have an MRI scan that shows us this cavum septum pellucidum, cavum vergae, bilateral hippocampal atrophy, and patchy, asymmetric atrophy of the left anterior temporal and frontal lobes.

Functional Imaging in CTE

Fig. 9.17 shows her FDG PET scan. Previously I showed you FDG PET scans (or analogous SPECT scans) of Alzheimer's disease (Fig. 9.6), dementia with Lewy bodies (Fig. 9.12), and frontotemporal dementia (Fig. 9.15). Let's keep those images in mind when we look at her scan. Fig. 9.17A and B shows that she has bilateral anterior and medial temporal lobe hypometabolism, but left is worse than right. Fig. 9.17C shows a

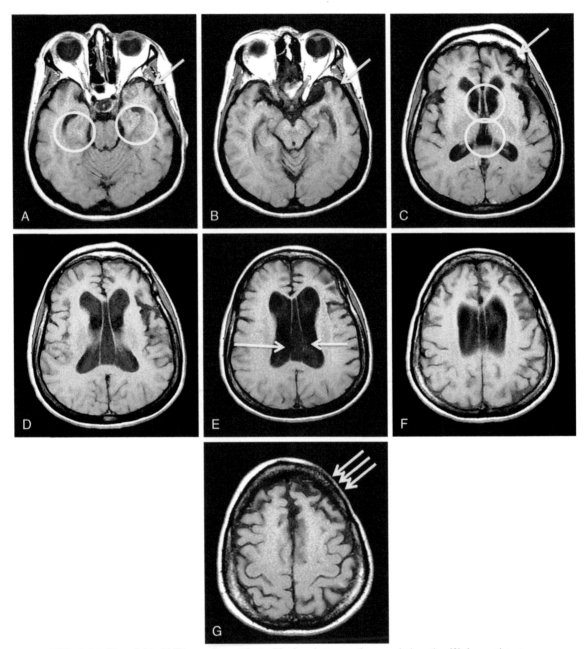

FIG. 9.16 T1-weighted MRI scan in a patient with chronic traumatic encephalopathy. (**A**) *Arrow* shows focal left anterior temporal lobe atrophy, *circles* show hippocampal atrophy. (**B**) *Arrow* shows focal left anterior temporal lobe atrophy. (**C**) *Arrow* shows focal left frontal atrophy. *Top circle* shows cavum septum pellucidum; *bottom circle* shows cavum vergae. (**D**) Cavum septum pellucidum and cavum vergae. (**E**) Cavum septum pellucidum and cavum vergae with multiple fenestrations at the level of the *arrows*. (**F**) Cavum and atrophy. (**G**) Focal left frontal atrophy (*arrows*). (Note that left side of brain is right side of image.)

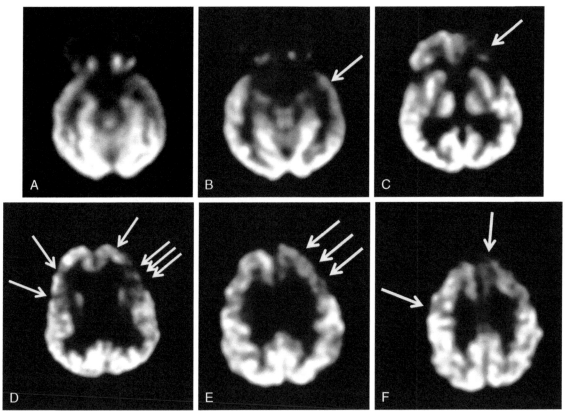

FIG. 9.17 A fluorodeoxyglucose PET scan shows (**A** and **B**) left > right medial and anterior temporal lobe hypometabolism, (**C**) focal left > right frontal hypometabolism, (**D**) patchy left > right frontal hypometabolism, (**E**) focal left > right frontal hypometabolism, and (**F**) left anterior cingulate gyrus and other regions of focal hypometabolism. (Note that left side of brain is right side of image.)

very asymmetric hypometabolism—the right side of the brain is doing pretty well, but the metabolism in left frontal lobe is greatly diminished. Fig. 9.17D shows a big patch of hypometabolism in the left frontal lobe and smaller patches of hypometabolism in the right frontal lobe. When I look at this image, I feel like I can infer some of the pathology that we have been looking at—you can almost see the pathology involving individual sulci producing this patchiness. Fig. 9.17E and F shows you more of this patchiness of the hypometabolism.

Clinical Diagnosis of Probable CTE

We made the diagnosis of probable CTE in this patient based on the combination of the clinical symptoms along with the MRI scan showing cavum septum pellucidum, cavum vergae, fenestrations of the septum, bilateral atrophy of the hippocampi and hypometabolism of the medial temporal lobes, and focal, patchy

areas of atrophy and hypometabolism in the cortex. See Box 9.8 for the research criteria for traumatic encephalopathy syndrome and Box 9.9 for potential biomarkers. Note that I have adapted these research criteria for clinical use.

Why do we have so many focal and patchy areas of cortical atrophy and hypometabolism? My guess is that it is directly related to the patchiness of the pathology. Why do we have more symmetric atrophy of hippocampi? My guess is because, as the disease progresses, both hippocampi become involved from hippocampal-cortical connections. Furthermore, as we have heard about the last day and a half, the regional distribution of the pathology is likely directly related to where the brain impacts were located. I want to show you a video of what she looked like when I saw her a year ago. I am still following her and she is still living, so I don't have a pathologic diagnosis on her, but for all the reasons

---

BOX 9.8
Criteria for Traumatic Encephalopathy Syndrome

General Criteria for Traumatic Encephalopathy Syndrome: *All five criteria must be met*

1. History of multiple impacts to the head based upon the type of injury (a) and source of exposure (b).

    a. Types of injuries:

        i. Mild traumatic brain injuries or concussions, minimum of four

        ii. Moderate/severe traumatic brain injury

        iii. "Subconcussive" trauma

    b. Source of exposures:

        i. Involvement of "high-exposure" contact sports for minimum of 6 years, including at least two at college level or higher

        ii. Military service

        iii. History of any other significant exposure to repetitive hits to the head

2. For moderate/severe traumatic brain injury, any activity resulting in the injury

3. No other neurological disorder present that likely accounts for all clinical features

4. Clinical features must be present for a minimum of 12 months

5. At least one Core Clinical Feature must be present and considered a change from baseline

6. At least two Supportive Features must be present

Core Clinical Features of Traumatic Encephalopathy Syndrome: *At least one must be met*

1. *Cognitive.* Difficulties in cognition as reported by either self or informant, by history, or clinician's report of decline *and* substantiated by impairment on standardized tests

2. *Behavioral.* Emotionally explosive, physically and/or verbally violent

3. *Mood.* Feeling overly sad, depressed, and/or hopeless

Supportive Features of Traumatic Encephalopathy Syndrome: *At least two must be present*

1. *Impulsivity.* Impaired impulse control as demonstrated by new behaviors

2. *Anxiety.* History of anxious mood, agitation, excessive fears, or obsessive and/or compulsive behavior

3. *Apathy.* Loss of interest in usual activities, loss of motivation and emotions, and/or reduction of voluntary, goal-directed behaviors

4. *Paranoia.* Delusional beliefs of suspicion, persecution, and/or unwarranted jealousy

5. *Suicidality.* History of suicidal thoughts or attempts

6. *Headache.* Significant and chronic headache, with at least one episode per month for 6 months

7. *Motor signs.* Dysarthria, dysgraphia, bradykinesia, tremor, rigidity, gait disturbance, falls, and/or other features of parkinsonism

8. *Documented decline.* Progressive decline in function and/or a progression in symptoms and/or signs, for a minimum of 1 year

9. *Delayed onset.* Delayed onset of clinical features after significant head impact exposure, usually at least 2 years and in many cases several years after the period of maximal exposure

Traumatic encephalopathy syndrome diagnostic subtypes: (1) Behavioral/Mood Variant, (2) Cognitive Variant, (3) Mixed Variant, (4) Dementia

Criteria for (4) Traumatic Encephalopathy Syndrome Dementia:

1. Progressive course of Cognitive Core Features, with or without Behavioral and/or Mood Core Features

2. Cognitive impairment (or cognitive impairment exacerbated by behavioral and/or mood) severe enough to interfere with the ability to function independently at work or in usual activities, including hobbies, and instrumental activities of daily living

Adapted from Montenigro PH, Baugh CM, Daneshvar DH, et al. Clinical subtypes of chronic traumatic encephalopathy: literature review and proposed research diagnostic criteria for traumatic encephalopathy syndrome. *Alzheimer's Research and Therapy.* 2014;6(5):68.

I just mentioned I am pretty sure that we have the right diagnosis. (Video 13. 1 from Budson and Solomon, 2016,[1] was reviewed.)

Pharmacological Treatment of Patients With Possible CTE

So how do we treat this patient and those like her? Depending upon the specific signs and symptoms that she has, we can try all the medications that we talked about thus far.

So, let's say that you have a patient that you suspect has CTE—perhaps they meet the criteria for traumatic encephalopathy syndrome—and they have a memory impairment as their major problem. In that case, I would try a cholinesterase inhibitor to see if it helps.

Let's say we have a different patient, a younger one, and his main problem is depression or anxiety or behavioral problems—let's say he meets the criteria for the behavioral/mood variant of traumatic encephalopathy syndrome—I would start with an SSRI

BOX 9.9
Potential Biomarkers for the Diagnosis of Probable Chronic Traumatic Encephalopathy

1. *Cavum septum pellucidum.* Or cavum vergae, or fenestrations based on neuroimaging study
2. Normal β-amyloid CSF levels
3. Elevated CSF p-tau/tau ratio
4. Negative amyloid imaging
5. *Cortical atrophy* beyond expected for age as seen on MRI (or CT), and in particular, frontal, thalamic, hippocampal, and/or amygdalar atrophy
6. *Positive tau imaging (experimental).* PET paired helical filament tau imaging suggestive of abnormal tau deposition
7. Cortical thinning (experimental). Based on MRI measurement

Adapted from Montenigro PH, Baugh CM, Daneshvar DH, et al. Clinical subtypes of chronic traumatic encephalopathy: literature review and proposed research diagnostic criteria for traumatic encephalopathy syndrome. *Alzheimer's Research and Therapy.* 2014;6(5):68.

---

antidepressant medication, either sertraline or escitalopram, as I described.

If there is explosivity and violent behavior and you have tried SSRI and it is still not helping, I would probably try an atypical neuroleptic such as risperidone. My urgency in trying something like an atypical neuroleptic would depend on how dangerous their behavior was. For example, if their family was afraid of them I would try it right away. You could also try the combination pill dextromethorphan/quinidine (Nuedexta) for the agitation.

If the individual is in the moderate to severe dementia stage, you can try memantine. Memantine was helpful in this patient I described. If there is pseudobulbar affect, you can try the combination pill dextromethorphan/quinidine (Nuedexta).

Nonpharmacological Treatment of Patients With Possible CTE

What about nonpharmacological things that one can do?

Aerobic exercise is very important—not only can it improve cardiovascular fitness, but also there are studies that show it can actually increase the size of the hippocampus in young healthy individuals by increasing new brain cells because aerobic exercise causes brain growth factors to be released. There are also many studies in older individuals that show even walking just 30 min a day, 5 days a week, can be beneficial.

Social activities and social interaction is also critically important—we don't want our patients to become isolated.

Regarding diets, the Mediterranean diet is really the only diet or food modification that has any evidence going for it, and I am pleased to say that every time a new study comes out about the Mediterranean diet it is always showing some benefits.

People always wonder, "should I do crossword puzzles or play Sudoku?" The data on this topic are very clear. They show that if you do crossword puzzles or play Sudoku you get better at crossword puzzles or Sudoku. There is currently no evidence that practicing these activities or playing computer games or doing computerized memory training or similar activities translate into general improvement in cognitive function—but having said that, there is no doubt it is better to do these things than to watch TV!

So, in summary, I hope that you now feel better equipped to diagnose and treat a patient who walks into your clinic with possible CTE. Thank you very much for your attention.

DISCLOSURES

Royalties from Elsevier Publishing for Budson AE & Solomon PR, Memory Loss, Alzheimer's Disease, and Dementia: A Practical Guide for Clinicians, 2016. Royalties from Oxford Univ. Press for Budson AE & O'Connor MK, Seven Steps to Managing Your Memory: What's Normal, What's Not, and What to Do About It, 2017. Speaker for Eli Lilly. Consultant for General Electric. Clinical trial investigator for Biogen, Eli Lilly, vTv therapeutics, Axovant.

REFERENCES

1. Budson AE, Solomon PR. *Memory Loss, Alzheimer's Disease, and Dementia: A Practical Guide for Clinicians.* 2nd ed. Elsevier; 2016. ISBN-10: 0323286615, ISBN-13: 978-0323286619.
2. Littlejohns TJ, Henley WE, Lang IA, et al. Vitamin D and the risk of dementia and Alzheimer disease. *Neurology.* 2014;83:920–928.
3. McKhann GM, Knopman DS, Chertkow H, et al. The diagnosis of dementia due to Alzheimer's disease: recommendations from the National Institute on Aging-Alzheimer's Association workgroups on diagnostic guidelines for Alzheimer's disease. *Alzheimer's and Dementia.* 2011;7:263–269.
4. Sperling RA, Aisen PS, Beckett LA, et al. Toward defining the preclinical stages of Alzheimer's disease: recommendations from the National Institute on Aging—Alzheimer's Association workgroups on diagnostic guidelines for Alzheimer's disease. *Alzheimer's and Dementia.* 2011;7:280–292.

5. Winblad B, Engedal K, Soininen H, et al. A 1-year, randomized, placebo-controlled study of donepezil in patients with mild to moderate AD. *Neurology*. August 14, 2001;57(3):489–495. PMID: 11502918.

6. Mohs RC, Doody RS, Morris JC, et al. A 1-year, placebo-controlled preservation of function survival study of donepezil in AD patients. *Neurology*. August 14, 2001;57(3):481–488. Erratum in: Neurology. November 27, 2001;57(10):1942. PMID: 11502917.

7. Trinh NH, Hoblyn J, Mohanty S, Yaffe K. Efficacy of cholinesterase inhibitors in the treatment of neuropsychiatric symptoms and functional impairment in Alzheimer disease: a meta-analysis. *JAMA*. January 8, 2003;289(2):210–216. Review. PMID: 12517232.

8. Howard R, McShane R, Lindesay J, et al. Donepezil and memantine for moderate-to-severe Alzheimer's disease. *The New England Journal of Medicine*. March 8, 2012;366(10):893–903. http://dx.doi.org/10.1056/NEJMoa1106668. PMID: 22397651.

9. Petersen RC, Thomas RG, Grundman M, et al. Vitamin E and donepezil for the treatment of mild cognitive impairment. *The New England Journal of Medicine*. June 9, 2005;352(23):2379–2388. PMID: 15829527.

10. McKeith IG, Dickson DW, Lowe J, et al. Diagnosis and management of dementia with Lewy bodies: third report of the DLB Consortium. *Neurology*. 2005;65:1863–1872.

11. McKeith I, Del Ser T, Spano P, et al. Efficacy of rivastigmine in dementia with Lewy bodies: a randomised, double-blind, placebo-controlled international study. *Lancet*. December 16, 2000;356(9247):2031–2036. PMID: 11145488.

12. Sachdev P, Kalaria R, O'Brien J, et al. Diagnostic criteria for vascular cognitive disorders: a VASCOG statement. *Alzheimer Disease and Associated Disorders*. 2014;28:206–218.

13. Roman GC, Wilkinson DG, Doody RS, et al. Donepezil in vascular dementia: combined analysis of two large-scale clinical trials. *Dementia and Geriatric Cognitive Disorders*. 2005;20:338–344.

14. Wilcock G, Mobius HJ, Stoffler A. A double-blind, placebo-controlled multicentre study of memantine in mild to moderate vascular dementia (MMM500). *International Clinical Psychopharmacology*. 2002;17:297–305.

15. Relkin N, Marmarou A, Klinge P, et al. Diagnosing idiopathic normal-pressure hydrocephalus. *Neurosurgery*. 2005;57:S4–S16.

16. Cummings JL, Lyketsos CG, Peskind ER, et al. Effect of dextromethorphan-quinidine on agitation in patients with Alzheimer disease dementia: a randomized clinical trial. *JAMA*. September 22–29, 2015;314(12):1242–1254. http://dx.doi.org/10.1001/jama.2015.10214. PMID: 26393847.

17. LaMarre AK, Rascovsky K, Bostrom A, et al. Interrater reliability of the new criteria for behavioral variant frontotemporal dementia. *Neurology*. 2013;80:1973–1977.

18. Montenigro PH, Baugh CM, Daneshvar DH, et al. Clinical subtypes of chronic traumatic encephalopathy: literature review and proposed research diagnostic criteria for traumatic encephalopathy syndrome. *Alzheimer's Research and Therapy*. 2014;6:68.

19. Rascovsky K, Hodges JR, Knopman D, et al. Sensitivity of revised diagnostic criteria for the behavioural variant of frontotemporal dementia. *Brain*. 2011;134:2456–2477.

Fluid Biomarkers for Mild Traumatic Brain Injury and Chronic Traumatic Encephalopathy

KAJ BLENNOW

INTRODUCTION

Thank you for inviting me here. It has been two very interesting, passionate, and fun days. I work in the clinic in neurochemistry in Gothenburg. It is a combined clinical and research lab, so we do a lot of clinical assays on cerebrospinal fluid (CSF) for Alzheimer's disease (AD) and several other diseases. Because of some of the similarities in pathology between AD and chronic traumatic encephalopathy (CTE) we became interested in studies of brain trauma.

An important question to start with is: why do we need biomarkers for traumatic brain injury (TBI), CTE, and the other diseases we are talking about? First, of course, is to aid in clinical diagnosis. Biomarkers can help to identify or rule out signs of neuronal damage and other types of pathophysiology. They can also be a guide to clinical management of these patients, for example, whether patients need a CT scan or not. Second, biomarkers may help to determine the severity of damage. Grading the severity of damage may help to predict prognosis, guide when contact sport athletes (such as boxers) should return to play, and guide the management of patients that have long-term postconcussion symptoms. Third, regarding drug development, biomarkers are important to monitor the effect on pathophysiology of novel drug candidates or other treatments. The importance of this type of monitoring has been clearly shown in AD because, like CTE, it is a slowly progressive disorder and difficult to stage by the symptoms alone, while biomarkers provide objective measures of the pathology and pathophysiology. Lastly, biomarkers are critical in clinical research studies in order to link pathophysiology directly to clinical signs and symptoms in patients, which will help us to understand more about TBI, CTE, postconcussion syndrome, and related disorders.[1]

So what options for biomarkers do we have? In Fig. 10.1 you can see a number of different potential biomarkers that are possible to measure in CSF, such as neuronal proteins, tau proteins, and also another axonal protein called neurofilament light. We can also measure synaptic proteins, β-amyloid (Aβ), the amyloid precursor protein, and a number of proteins from astrocytes, as well as inflammatory proteins and even some proteins in the dendrites. So there are a number of possible candidates, but since neurons are the functional units of the brain, we believe that axonal proteins may be the best ones, such as neurofilament light and tau proteins.[2]

CEREBRAL SPINAL FLUID BIOMARKERS

I will start by describing some studies in which we measured biomarkers in CSF. CSF is fluid produced in the brain by filtration from the plasma and from the brain bidirectionally (Fig. 10.2). Thus, the composition of CSF reflects brain biochemistry. CSF flows out from the ventricles and into the subarachnoid space, and part of it diffuses down along the spinal cord, so you can obtain CSF by performing a lumbar puncture (LP) in the lower back region. I would like to note that an LP is a routine procedure in clinical medicine commonly used for diagnosis of disorders such as meningitis, multiple sclerosis, and AD, as well as for administration of spinal anesthesia. The frequency of a post-LP headache is below 10%, and almost always mild, while serious complications (such as meningitis, paresis, hematoma) are rare.[3] Post-LP headaches are less common if smaller and nontraumatic needles are used, and they are also less common in older individuals.

Acute TBI

Another way to obtain CSF is from the brain ventricles, and this you can do in patients with severe brain trauma that have a ventricular catheter in place to reduce intracranial pressure (Fig. 10.3). Daily ventricular CSF

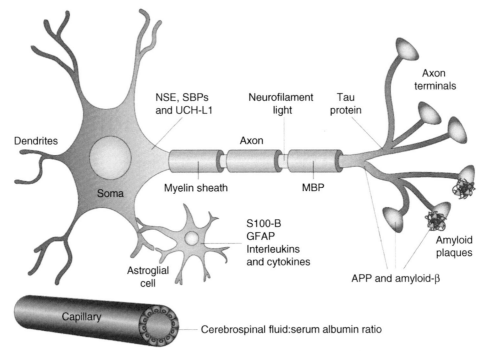

FIG. 10.1 Candidate biomarkers of mild traumatic brain injury in cerebrospinal fluid and blood. *APP*, amyloid precursor protein; *GFAP*, glial fibrillary acidic protein; *MBP*, myelin basic protein; *NFL*, neurofilament light; *NSE*, neuron-specific enolase; *SBP*, spectrin breakdown products; *UCHL1*, ubiquitin carboxyl-terminal hydrolase L1. (From Zetterberg H, Smith DH, Blennow K. Biomarkers of mild traumatic brain injury in cerebrospinal fluid and blood. *Nature Reviews. Neurology.* April 2013;9(4):201–210. http://dx.doi.org/10.1038/nrneurol.2013.9.)

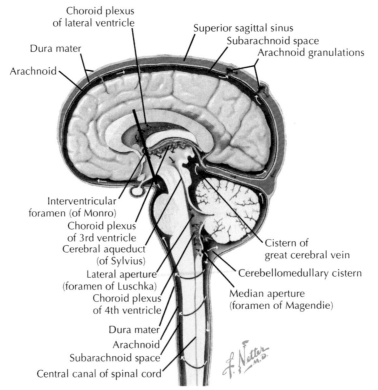

FIG. 10.2 The production of cerebrospinal fluid. (Netter illustration from www.netterimages.com. Copyright Elsevier Inc. All rights reserved.)

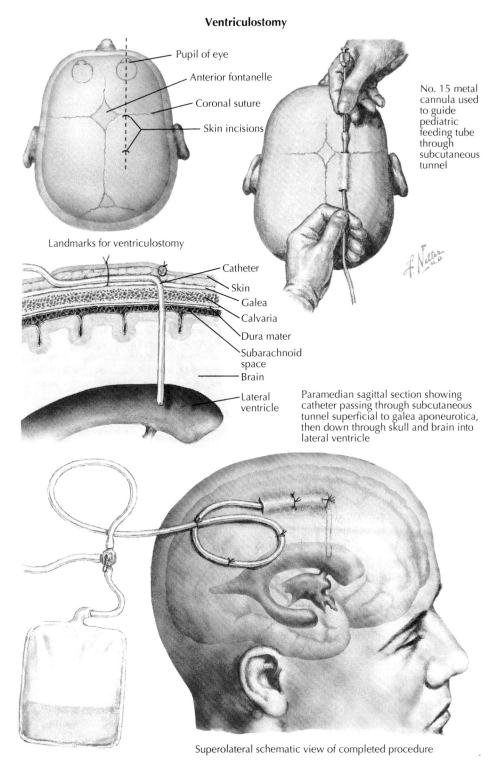

Ventriculostomy

- Pupil of eye
- Anterior fontanelle
- Coronal suture
- Skin incisions

Landmarks for ventriculostomy

No. 15 metal cannula used to guide pediatric feeding tube through subcutaneous tunnel

- Catheter
- Skin
- Galea
- Calvaria
- Dura mater
- Subarachnoid space
- Brain
- Lateral ventricle

Paramedian sagittal section showing catheter passing through subcutaneous tunnel superficial to galea aponeurotica, then down through skull and brain into lateral ventricle

Superolateral schematic view of completed procedure

FIG. 10.3 Obtaining ventricular cerebrospinal fluid samples. (Netter illustration from www.netterimages.com. Copyright Elsevier Inc. All rights reserved.)

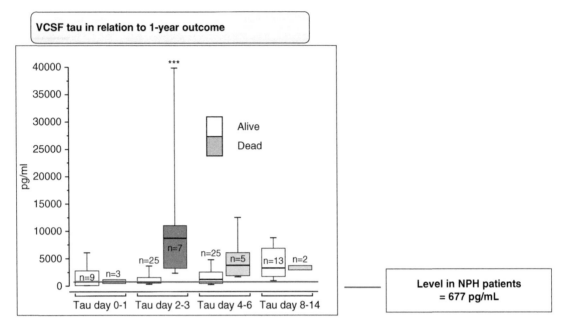

FIG. 10.4 Initial cerebrospinal fluid (CSF) total tau correlates with 1-year outcome in patients with traumatic brain injury (TBI). A marked increase in ventricular CSF (VCSF) tau after acute severe TBI predicts a lower likelihood of survival. As a comparison, the *red line* shows the level of total tau in the ventricular CSF of patients with normal-pressure hydrocephalus (NPH). (From Öst M, Nylén K, Csajbok L, et al. Initial CSF total tau correlates with 1-year outcome in patients with traumatic brain injury. *Neurology*. November 14, 2006;67(9):1600–1604.)

sampling is possible in severe TBI cases with ventricular catheters and may aid in identifying biomarker candidates. Fig. 10.4 shows the results of a study measuring total tau in patients with acute brain trauma.[4] You can see that around days 2 and 3 tau increased tremendously—about 10-fold—in those patients with poor prognoses. Similarly, CSF neurofilament light shows elevations starting at days 0 to 2 and persisting throughout days 11 to 18 in those with a worse prognosis after acute TBI (Fig. 10.5).[5] One difference between measuring total tau and neurofilament light in the CSF is that, whereas total tau was only elevated in those who had very severe TBI, neurofilament light also increased in those patients with more moderate TBIs compared to normal-pressure hydrocephalus patients as controls. Thus, neurofilament light shows more promise as a biomarker for TBI compared to tau.

Boxers

We did a study on amateur boxers who underwent two LPs, the first 7 to 10 days after a bout and the second after 3 months of rest. Although we measured six different CSF biomarkers, only neurofilament light showed a clear difference in CSF levels for three key comparisons: between boxers after a bout versus after rest, between boxers after a bout versus control subjects, and between boxers after rest versus control subjects.[6] Not only that, we also found that neurofilament light showed the highest levels in those boxers who had many hits compared to those with few hits (Fig. 10.6). You can see the marked increase right after a bout and how the levels go back almost to normal after rest.

We did a follow-up study with help from the Swedish Boxing Association with 30 boxers and 25 controls. We obtained two CSF samples, one shortly after a bout and then again at a follow-up time after rest. In this study, we saw a very similar marked increase in neurofilament light in 25 of 30 boxers (83%) after a bout and a persistent increase in 13 of those 25 (52%) at the follow-up LP. Again there was a correlation between the boxing exposure score and the level of neurofilament light (Fig. 10.7).[7] Other proteins were also measured, and although there was some change in tau and S-100B, it was very minor, so we think that neurofilament light is the most promising candidate as a biomarker for concussion.

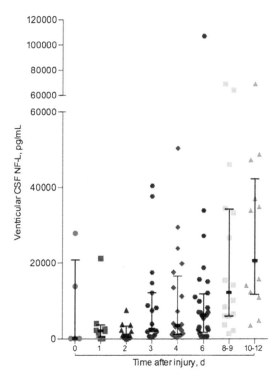

FIG. 10.5 Cerebrospinal fluid (CSF) neurofilament light protein after acute traumatic brain injury. (From Shahim P, Gren M, Liman V, et al. Serum neurofilament light protein predicts clinical outcome in traumatic brain injury. *Scientific Reports*. November 7, 2016;6:36791. http://dx.doi.org/10.1 038/srep36791.)

Window of Vulnerability Hypothesis

One hypothesis that many people have been considering is the window of vulnerability. In short, it means that the pathophysiological processes that occur after a TBI take time to resolve and return to normal. If you have a new hit to the head prior to resolution of the prior damage it might be worse than if you allowed the brain to fully recover (Fig. 10.8).[8-10]

We were actually contacted by a boxer who knew of our work and the vulnerability hypothesis who wanted us to study him so that he would know when it was safe for him to go back into the ring. He was knocked out during a bout and was unconscious for maybe 5 min. He asked us for an LP—this is not common! When we found his level of neurofilament light was highly elevated he asked for another LP, and another, until his levels returned to normal. As you can see in Fig. 10.9, it took more than 28 weeks for his CSF neurofilament light level to return to the normal

range.[11] Although this is one single case, these findings support that fluid biomarkers may guide return-to-play decisions.

Soccer Players

After these studies showing the brain injury biomarkers in boxers began to come out, the Swedish Boxing Association wrote to several newspapers, including the Swedish medical journal *Dagens Medicin* (English: Medicine Today) criticizing our work and stating that these biomarkers must also be elevated in other sports such as soccer. So we did the following study with 23 soccer players and 9 control students. The players needed to head the ball to the kicker 30 m away and they were asked to do either 10 or 20 approved headings (ball headed properly and going in the correct direction toward the kicker). This task was a difficult one for the players. We tested their CSF 1 week later for neurofilament light, total tau, glial fibrillary acidic protein (GFAP), and S-100B. There were no differences in any measures between the soccer players and controls—all of the players had neurofilament light levels below 125 ng/L.[12] So, in short, there were no changes suggestive of alteration of the blood-brain barrier or damage to the brain. When you are heading the ball in soccer, you have tensed the muscles in your neck, so that when your head meets the ball your head doesn't move, then the brain won't rotate. It's like standing with your back against the wall and someone shoots a ball straight to your forehead; it will bounce off without causing any rotation of the head. By contrast, in boxing when you get hit in the head your head rotates and accelerates in many different ways.

BLOOD-BASED BIOMARKERS
S-100B

Of course, it would be much easier if we could do blood sampling instead of LPs. It is like the Holy Grail for TBI biomarkers. In Europe, some groups have suggested the S-100B protein and they have written guidelines for the initial management of TBI.[13] In short, there are a number of studies showing that S-100B has a good sensitivity (97%) to detect intracranial complications such as hemorrhages, such that it may reduce the need to obtain a CT scan. So, if you do an S-100B test and it is normal, you don't have to do the scan, but, on the other hand, it has very low specificity (34%), so you will have many false positives. The reason for the low specificity is that S-100B is also present in some other organs of the body, meaning that peripheral trauma will also result in increased S-100B levels. In addition, a study

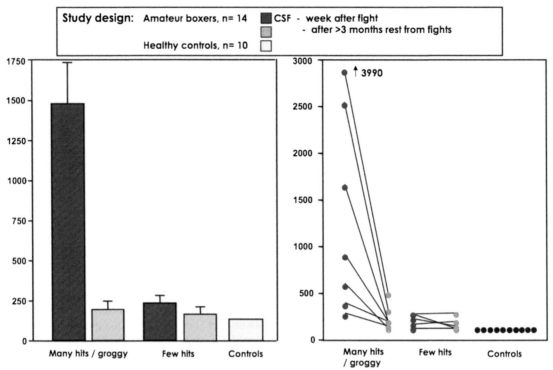

FIG. 10.6 Cerebrospinal fluid (CSF) neurofilament light in boxers. (From Zetterberg H, Hietala MA, Jonsson M, et al. Neurochemical aftermath of amateur boxing. *Archives of Neurology*. September 2006;63(9):1277–1280.)

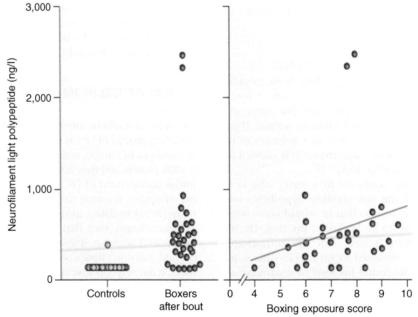

FIG. 10.7 Increase in the axonal protein neurofilament light in boxers after a bout. (From Neselius S, Brisby H, Theodorsson A, Blennow K, Zetterberg H, Marcusson J. CSF-biomarkers in Olympic boxing: diagnosis and effects of repetitive head trauma. *PLoS One*. 2012;7(4):e33606. http://dx.doi.org/10.1371/journal.pone.0033606.)

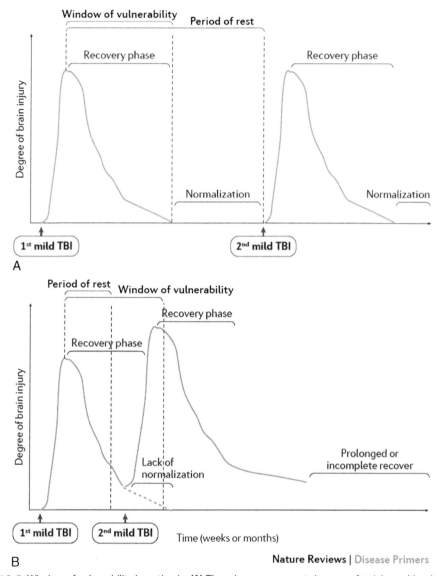

FIG. 10.8 Window of vulnerability hypothesis: **(A)** There is no permanent damage after injury with adequate recovery and rest periods. **(B)** Insufficient rest and recovery time can lead to prolonged or incomplete recovery. *TBI*, traumatic brain injury. (From Blennow K, Brody DL, Kochanek PM, et al. Traumatic brain injuries. *Nature Reviews Disease Primers*. November 17, 2016;2:16084. http://dx.doi.org/10.1038/nrdp.2016.84.)

in 2012 found that in patients with mild TBI there was actually no difference at all in S-100B between CT or MRI positive or negative hemorrhage cases and also no correlation with clinical outcomes.[14] So we clearly need better biomarkers than S-100B.

Single-Molecule Array in Serum and Plasma

As you know, the concentration of these neuronal proteins in the CSF is really low, and in the blood they are

even lower. For example, the tau concentration in CSF is 500 pg/mL, which is not much at all, and in blood it is only 5 pg/mL. To help you visualize this quantity, 5 pg/mL is like detecting one-hundredth of a sugar cube in an Olympic size pool—after you add in 40 tons of other proteins—and you need to be able to measure a 10% or 20% difference. There is a new technique called single-molecule array (Simoa) that can measure from 0.025 to 250 pg/mL.[15] In short, this assay is similar to those based

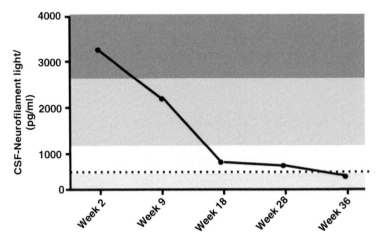

FIG. 10.9 Monitoring concussion in a knocked-out boxer by cerebrospinal fluid (CSF) neurofilament light (NFL). (From Neselius S, Brisby H, Granholm F, Zetterberg H, Blennow K. Monitoring concussion in a knocked-out boxer by CSF biomarker analysis. *Knee Surgery, Sports Traumatology, Arthroscopy.* September 2015;23(9):2536–2539. http://dx.doi.org/10.1007/s00167-014-3066-6.)

on magnetic beads that are coated with antibodies and the immunoreaction takes place on the bead surface. However, instead of measuring the total fluorescence, each bead fits into a small microwell, and, in the end, you measure the ratio between positive and negative beads. This technique can provide really good analytical sensitivity. For example, using an assay for tau that we worked on together with the company who developed it, the sensitivity was 0.02 pg/mL, which is 1000 times better than the standard enzyme-linked immunosorbent assay (ELISA) method and also has a very wide analytical range.

Plasma Tau in Ice Hockey Players
We started with a study on ice hockey players using tau in blood. In the highest league in Sweden, 45 players got a concussion during the 2012-2013 season. We had the teams draw blood after concussion at 1 h, 12 h, 36 h, 6 days, and return to play. Although there was not a clear increase in plasma tau in relation to the severity of the symptoms, there was a correlation between the 1-h plasma tau levels and the return to play time.[15]

Plasma Tau as a Marker for Concussion in Boxers
We did the same thing with 30 Olympic boxers and 25 controls, measuring tau and other brain proteins in their blood 1 to 6 days after a bout and then again after more than 14 days of rest. We found a mild increase in plasma tau in boxers after a bout (2.46 pg/mL) that decreased after rest (1.43 pg/mL), although not back to the levels of controls (0.79 pg/mL). There was, however, quite a lot of overlap between the results of the boxers and controls. Note that there was no change in any other protein such as S-100B, GFAP, Aβ, or brain derived neurotrophic factor levels in this study.[17]

Measuring Neurofilament Light in Serum and Plasma
I have also been working on measuring neurofilament light in serum and plasma using the Simoa technique.[18] In short, although both ELISA and Simoa work to measure neurofilament light in CSF, only Simoa has the sensitivity required to measure neurofilament light in serum and plasma. Importantly, we have now compared CSF and blood samples for neurofilament light in five different cohorts, and the correlation between them is really tight, in the range of r equaling about 0.85 to 0.90 (Fig. 10.10). So now, more or less, you can replace CSF sampling with blood sampling if you are going to measure neurofilament light.

Serum Neurofilament Light and S-100B in Patients With Acute, Severe TBI
We conducted a study on 70 patients with acute, severe TBI and 35 age-matched controls and measured neurofilament light and S-100B. Fig. 10.11 shows that neurofilament light started elevated at the first time point and also showed a very marked increase starting around 6 days up to around 12 days, mostly returning to normal in the patients that survived after 1 year. S-100B also shows an increase at the first time point and day 1, returning mostly to normal after day 2.[19] It is important to note that the time course for these biomarkers is different.

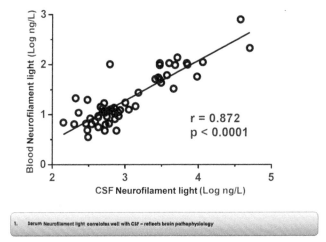

FIG. 10.10 Neurofilament light (NFL) in cerebrospinal fluid (CSF) versus blood in patients with human immunodeficiency virus infection with varying severity of central nervous system involvement. (Figure from Gisslén M, Price RW, Andreasson U, et al. Plasma concentration of the neurofilament light protein (NFL) is a biomarker of CNS injury in HIV infection: a cross-sectional study. *EBioMedicine*. November 22, 2015;3:135–140. http://dx.doi.org/10.1016/j.ebiom.2015.11.036. PMID: 26870824.)

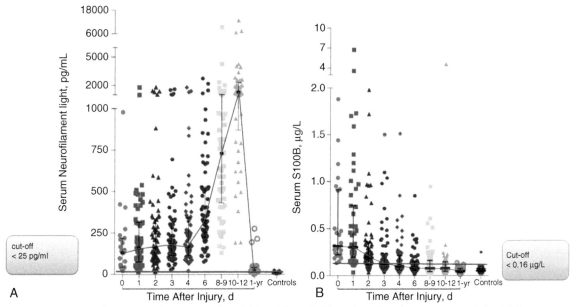

FIG. 10.11 Serum neurofilament light (NF-L) **(A)** and S-100B **(B)** as biomarkers for acute traumatic brain injury. (Modified from Shahim P, Gren M, Liman V, et al. Serum neurofilament light protein predicts clinical outcome in traumatic brain injury. *Scientific Reports*. November 7, 2016;6:36791. http://dx.doi.org/10.1038/srep36791.)

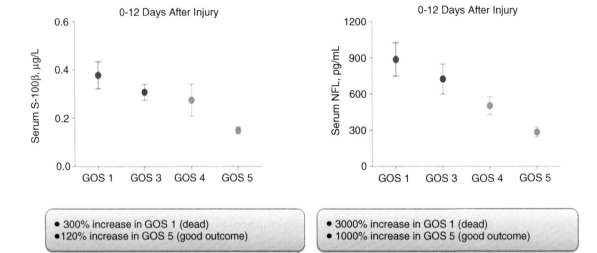

FIG. 10.12 Comparison between serum neurofilament light **(A)** and S-100B **(B)** as prognostic markers in acute traumatic brain injury (TBI). Serum neurofilament light, but not S-100B, predicts 1-year function outcome in patients with TBI. (Modified from Shahim P, Gren M, Liman V, et al. Serum neurofilament light protein predicts clinical outcome in traumatic brain injury. *Scientific Reports*. November 7, 2016;6:36791. http://dx.doi.org/10.1038/srep36791.)

Fig. 10.12 shows that there was also a correlation with clinical outcome at 1 year. Compared to control levels, there was a 3000% increase for those who died versus 1000% increase even for those who had a good outcome. By contrast, for S-100B you don't have a clear change. In short, we believe that blood neurofilament light would be a good biomarker for TBI.

Serum Neurofilament Light in Amateur Boxers

We measured serum neurofilament light in 14 amateur boxers compared to 12 age-matched controls and 12 gymnasts as an athletic control group. We found that 7 to 10 days after a bout serum neurofilament light increases, and after 3 months rest it decreases, but not down to the level of controls. We also found that the relative increase in serum neurofilament light varies with the severity of the head impact.[20] So, in summary, neurofilament light correlates with the severity of brain damage and can be measured in the serum. I believe this marker is the best candidate as a blood biomarker for concussion.

BIOMARKERS FOR POSTCONCUSSIVE SYNDROME

Hockey Players

How about we now take a look not at the acute injury but go a bit later to evaluate those with postconcussion syndrome who have persistent symptoms lasting at least for several months. In the Swedish professional hockey league there are a number of players who had to stop playing—they don't want to stop but they have to stop—because of postconcussive symptoms lasting different lengths of time. In this study, we met 9 players who had symptoms more than 1 year who couldn't play hockey and 7 with a shorter duration of symptoms and compared them to 15 controls. The players volunteered to undergo spinal taps and even paid for their flight tickets to Gothenburg. We interviewed them about their symptoms and how many concussions they had. Even after several months or more than a year since their last concussion there were a number of players with elevated neurofilament light levels in CSF. CSF neurofilament light also correlated with the Rivermead Post-Concussion Symptoms Questionnaire and the history of lifetime concussions.[21]

BIOMARKERS FOR REPETITIVE HEAD INJURY

Plasma Total Tau in National Football League Players

The next results that I will show are from the Diagnosing and Evaluating Traumatic Encephalopathy using Clinical Tests (DETECT) study led by Dr. Robert Stern (Chapter 3). Plasma tau was examined in 96 former National Football League (NFL) players and 25 age-matched controls. Each player had to have played in the NFL for at least two seasons and played football for

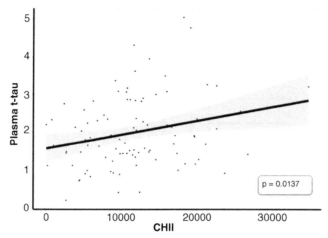

FIG. 10.13 Greater exposure to repetitive head impacts is associated with higher later-life plasma total tau, after adjustment for age and body mass index. Note that it is possible that those former players with extremely high total tau are starting to develop chronic traumatic encephalopathy pathology. (From Alosco ML, Tripodis Y, Jarnagin J, et al. Repetitive head impact exposure and later-life plasma total tau in former NFL players. 2017 [in press]. http://dx.doi.org/10.1016/j.dadm.2016.11.003.)

at least 12 years total, but could not have had a concussion for at least a year. Overall, there were no group differences in plasma total tau levels, but some former NFL players exhibited very high levels of plasma total tau (≥3.56 pg/mL), whereas no control subject had a level so high.[22] In addition, if you count head impacts using the cumulative head impact index (CHII), you can see correlations with plasma total tau levels after controlling for age and body mass index that were significant (Fig. 10.13), so plasma total tau levels may track the cumulative neural damage of repeated head impacts. Note that it is also possible that players with extremely high levels of total tau in their blood may be players who are starting to develop CTE pathology. We will have to see in the future if this hypothesis is correct.

Exosomal Tau in National Football League Players

Exosomes are small vesicles that are secreted from different tissues, including from the brain, into blood and CSF. These results are also from a published study by Dr. Stern and colleagues using the same players and controls as before. Here they isolated exosomes in blood and then measured different proteins including tau in the exosomes. It looks like a really promising technique. Fig. 10.14 shows higher tau levels in the NFL players compared with controls, with good sensitivity and specificity. You can see also that exosomal tau correlates with clinical measures including memory and psychomotor speed.[23] So exosomal tau and maybe also other proteins in exosomes are very promising potential biomarker candidates, although, of course, we need further studies.

Neurofilament Light in National Football League Players

How about examining neurofilament light in active NFL players? This work is a study we did together with Dr. Jonathan Oliver. We examined 20 NFL players over the course of a season divided into starters and nonstarters, with the thought that starters would have a higher exposure to head impact than nonstarters. Repeated blood samples were taken prior to the season and then at eight time points during the season. We used 20 swimmers as controls. Fig. 10.15 shows the results. You can see that over the course of the season neurofilament light in the serum slowly goes up, even though most of the impacts are subconcussive.[24]

We conducted a study that we did with Dr. Stern measuring plasma neurofilament light in his DETECT study cohort of 95 former NFL players and 22 age-matched controls. We did not find a real difference in absolute levels between groups and there was no correlation with CHII, but there were five former NFL players with very high levels of neurofilament light—greater than 35 pg/mL—that was higher than what was seen in any controls. We sometimes see this type of high level of neurofilament light in patients with neurodegenerative disorders, and so we will have to learn in the future whether these former NFL players have early CTE.

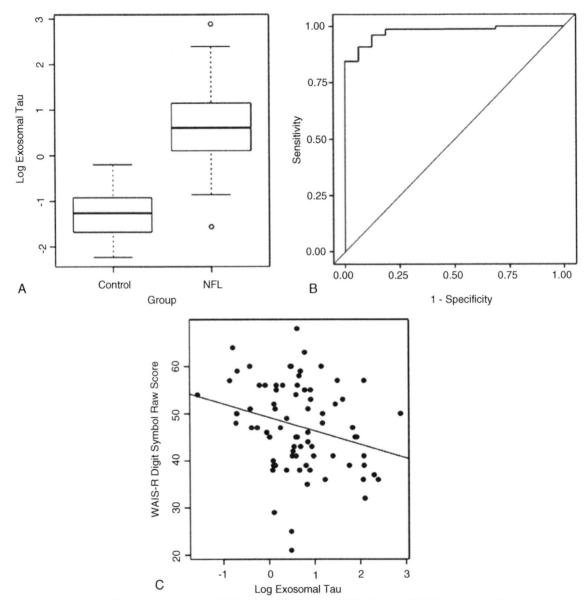

FIG. 10.14 Exosomal tau in former National Football League (NFL) players. **(A)** Higher exosomal tau present in former NFL players versus controls (P <.0001). **(B)** Compared with controls, sensitivity of exosomal tau to detect a former NFL player was 82%, specificity 100%. **(C)** Exosomal tau in correlates with psychomotor speed as measured by WAIS-R digit symbol raw score. (From Stern RA, Tripodis Y, Baugh CM, et al. Preliminary study of plasma exosomal tau as a potential biomarker for chronic traumatic encephalopathy. *The Journal of Alzheimer's Disease*. 2016;51(4):1099–1109. http://dx.doi.org/10.3233/JAD-151028.)

THE TIME COURSE OF CHANGE IN PLASMA BIOMARKERS IS KEY

In the future, it will be important to learn more about the time course of change for these biomarkers in head injury. Tau seems to be already elevated after 1 h, peaking around 6 h, and then going down at 1 day, although at 2 days it may be a bit elevated compared to baseline in some patients. Fig. 10.16 shows that S-100B peaks after 1 day and then slowly returns to baseline. Fig. 10.16 also shows neurofilament light, which goes up slowly after 2 to 3 days, peaks in the range of 1 to 2 weeks, and takes more than a month to return to baseline in many

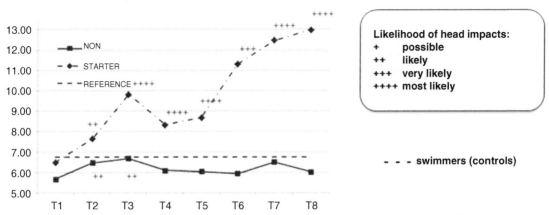

FIG. 10.15 Serum neurofilament light in National Football League players over the course of a season. (From Oliver JM, Jones MT, Kirk KM, et al. Serum neurofilament light in American football athletes over the course of a season. *Journal of Neurotrauma*. October 1, 2016;33(19):1784–1789.)

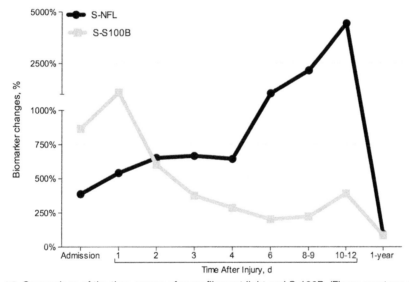

FIG. 10.16 Comparison of the time course of neurofilament light and S-100B. (Figure courtesy of Dr. Kaj Blennow.)

patients, with most patients showing normal levels after 1 year. When we looked at neurofilament light in stroke patients we found a similar pattern.

We are still learning about what happens with CSF and blood biomarkers after a TBI. Can we identify such biomarkers for CTE? We don't know the answer to that question, but we heard a lot about CTE in the past couple of days. CTE involves phosphorylated tau, neurodegeneration, and in some cases deposition of β-amyloid. We already have the CSF biomarkers neurofilament light, β-amyloid 42 and 40, phosphorylated tau, and total tau. We also have amyloid PET and tau PET. I think we need to wait for the longitudinal studies

on the suspected cases to learn whether these biomarkers will work to identify CTE.

The most important point that I will make today is also the last sentence that I managed to get into the abstract of a literature review paper on TBI and CTE that we just finished: Given that CTE is attributed to repeated head trauma, prevention might be possible through rule changes by sports organizations and legislators.[8] That's my take-home message from all this: Why do we accept boxing and why don't we demand rule changes in other sports, such as American football, that cause repeated concussions, when they can lead to this terrible disease?

DISCLOSURES

Dr. Blennow has served as a consultant or at advisory boards for Alzheon, Eli-Lilly, Fujirebio Europe, IBL International, and Roche Diagnostics and is a cofounder of Brain Biomarker Solutions in Gothenburg AB, a GU Venture-based platform company at the University of Gothenburg.

REFERENCES

1. Zetterberg H, Blennow K. Fluid biomarkers for mild traumatic brain injury and related conditions. *Nature Reviews. Neurology.* October 2016;12(10):563–574. http://dx.doi.org/10.1038/nrneurol.2016.127.

2. Zetterberg H, Smith DH, Blennow K. Biomarkers of mild traumatic brain injury in cerebrospinal fluid and blood. *Nature Reviews. Neurology.* April 2013;9(4):201–210. http://dx.doi.org/10.1038/nrneurol.2013.9.

3. Zetterberg H, Tullhög K, Hansson O, Minthon L, Londos E, Blennow K. Low incidence of post-lumbar puncture headache in 1,089 consecutive memory clinic patients. *European Neurology.* 2010;63(6):326–330. http://dx.doi.org/10.1159/000311703.

4. Öst M, Nylén K, Csajbok L, et al. Initial CSF total tau correlates with 1-year outcome in patients with traumatic brain injury. *Neurology.* November 14, 2006;67(9):1600–1604.

5. Shahim P, Gren M, Liman V, et al. Serum neurofilament light protein predicts clinical outcome in traumatic brain injury. *Scientific Reports.* 2016;6:36791.

6. Zetterberg H, Hietala MA, Jonsson M, et al. Neurochemical aftermath of amateur boxing. *Archives of Neurology.* September 2006;63(9):1277–1280.

7. Neselius S, Brisby H, Theodorsson A, Blennow K, Zetterberg H, Marcusson J. CSF-biomarkers in Olympic boxing: diagnosis and effects of repetitive head trauma. *PLoS One.* 2012;7(4):e33606. http://dx.doi.org/10.1371/journal.pone.0033606.

8. Blennow K, Brody DL, Kochanek PM, et al. Traumatic brain injuries. *Nature Reviews Disease Primers.* November 17, 2016;2:16084. http://dx.doi.org/10.1038/nrdp.2016.84.

9. Guskiewicz KM, McCrea M, Marshall SW, et al. Cumulative effects associated with recurrent concussion in collegiate football players: the NCAA Concussion Study. *JAMA.* November 19, 2003;290(19):2549–2555.

10. Slobounov S, Slobounov E, Sebastianelli W, Cao C, Newell K. Differential rate of recovery in athletes after first and second concussion episodes. *Neurosurgery.* August 2007;61(2):338–344. Discussion 344.

11. Neselius S, Brisby H, Granholm F, Zetterberg H, Blennow K. Monitoring concussion in a knocked-out boxer by CSF biomarker analysis. *Knee Surgery, Sports Traumatology, Arthroscopy.* September 2015;23(9):2536–2539. http://dx.doi.org/10.1007/s00167-014-3066-6.

12. Zetterberg H, Jonsson M, Rasulzada A, et al. No neurochemical evidence for brain injury caused by heading in soccer. *British Journal of Sports Medicine.* September 2007;41(9):574–577.

13. Undén J, Ingebrigtsen T, Romner B, Scandinavian Neurotrauma Committee (SNC). Scandinavian guidelines for initial management of minimal, mild and moderate head injuries in adults: an evidence and consensus-based update. *BMC Medicine.* February 25, 2013;11:50. http://dx.doi.org/10.1186/1741-7015-11-50.

14. Metting Z, Wilczak N, Rodiger LA, Schaaf JM, van der Naalt J. GFAP and S100B in the acute phase of mild traumatic brain injury. *Neurology.* May 1, 2012;78(18):1428–1433. http://dx.doi.org/10.1212/WNL.0b013e318253d5c7.

15. Randall J, Mörtberg E, Provuncher GK, et al. Tau proteins in serum predict neurological outcome after hypoxic brain injury from cardiac arrest: results of a pilot study. *Resuscitation.* March 2013;84(3):351–356. http://dx.doi.org/10.1016/j.resuscitation.2012.07.027.

16. Shahim P, Tegner Y, Wilson DH, et al. Blood biomarkers for brain injury in concussed professional ice hockey players. *JAMA Neurology.* June 2014;71(6):684–692.

17. Neselius S, Zetterberg H, Blennow K, Randall J, Wilson D, Marcusson J, Brisby H. Olympic boxing is associated with elevated levels of the neuronal protein tau in plasma. *Brain Injury.* 2013;27(4):425–433. http://dx.doi.org/10.3109/02699052.2012.750752.

18. Gisslén M, Price RW, Andreasson U, et al. Plasma concentration of the neurofilament light protein (NFL) is a biomarker of CNS injury in HIV Infection: a cross-sectional study. *EBioMedicine.* November 22, 2015;3:135–140. http://dx.doi.org/10.1016/j.ebiom.2015.11.036. PMID: 26870824.

19. Shahim P, Gren M, Liman V, et al. Serum neurofilament light protein predicts clinical outcome in traumatic brain injury. *Scientific Reports.* November 7, 2016a;6:36791. http://dx.doi.org/10.1038/srep36791.

20. Shahim P, Zetterberg H, Tegner Y, Blennow K. Serum neurofilament light as a biomarker for mild traumatic brain injury in contact sports. *Neurology.* 2017;88:1788–1794.

21. Shahim P, Tegner Y, Gustafsson B, et al. Neurochemical aftermath of repetitive mild traumatic brain injury. *JAMA Neurology.* November 1, 2016b;73(11):1308–1315. http://dx.doi.org/10.1001/jamaneurol.2016.2038.

22. Alosco ML, Tripodis Y, Jarnagin J, et al. Repetitive head impact exposure and later-life plasma total tau in former National Football League players. *Alzheimer's & Dementia.* 2016;7:33-40. http://dx.doi.org/10.1016/j.dadm.2016.11.003.

23. Stern RA, Tripodis Y, Baugh CM, et al. Preliminary study of plasma exosomal tau as a potential biomarker for chronic traumatic encephalopathy. *Journal of Alzheimer's Disease.* 2016;51(4):1099–1109. http://dx.doi.org/10.3233/JAD-151028.

24. Oliver JM, Jones MT, Kirk KM, et al. Serum neurofilament light in American football athletes over the course of a season. *Journal of Neurotrauma.* October 1, 2016;33(19):1784–1789.

CHAPTER 11

Toward Imaging Chronic Traumatic Encephalopathy

MARTHA E. SHENTON • INGA K. KOERTE

OVERVIEW

Today I will present collaborative work on chronic traumatic encephalopathy (CTE) that I have conducted with Dr. Robert Stern and colleagues, first as part of his R01 and now as part of our U01, both funded by the National Institutes of Health (NIH). I am a scientist at the Veterans Affairs (VA) Boston Healthcare System, and I am also at Brigham and Women's Hospital and Harvard Medical School. I have been a schizophrenia researcher for over 30 years, and what I find interesting about moving into what are new areas of research for me (CTE and mild traumatic brain injury [TBI]) are the differences and similarities in addressing questions about the brain.

What I learned from schizophrenia is that, when researching a brain disorder one needs to have the right methods in order to answer the questions one wants to have answered. We used sophisticated neuroimaging methodologies for our schizophrenia research and really nailed it as a brain disorder. We then began to use diffusion imaging, which brought us to thinking about brain injury, because one of the main injuries in mild TBI is diffuse axonal injury, which can be detected using diffusion magnetic resonance (MR) imaging. This again emphasized to us that the right methods are needed in order to answer the questions one wants to have answered.

By way of introduction I will quickly review the two NIH-funded studies, Diagnosing and Evaluating Traumatic Encephalopathy using Clinical Tests (DETECT) and Diagnostics, Imaging, and Genetics Network for the Objective Study and Evaluation (DIAGNOSE) of CTE (Chapter 3). We point out certain methodologies we are using, but will not discuss all of them in detail. We will next review the background of CTE and also brain imaging findings from our retired National Football League (NFL) players, beginning with case studies showing cortical atrophy and cavum septum pellucidum (CSP). Importantly, we will also show age-related changes and new unpublished data. We will also present imaging findings from subconcussive repetitive blows to the head in other sports such as soccer and ice hockey. We will then review data from the DETECT and DIAGNOSE CTE studies acquired thus far and some of the hopes that we have for these studies going forward.

Currently, the only way to diagnose CTE is by postmortem evaluation. In DETECT and DIAGNOSE, we are investigating individuals who have presumed CTE with the goal of developing diagnostic criteria in vivo. This is important because if one can make an in vivo diagnosis, then maybe one can intervene early in the illness, stop the progression, and maybe even one day prevent the disease entirely. In DETECT, we've been acquiring imaging and other measures on more than 96 NFL players, currently the largest number of retired NFL players who've ever been imaged.

Regarding MR methodologies, an important one is *morphometry*, parceling the brain into volumes and shapes. Think of it as measuring a cup: how full it is also tells one how empty it is. Shape is important for neurodevelopmental changes in the brain, particularly structures in the middle region of the brain, such as the corpus callosum. Other methodologies used in DETECT are diffusion MR imaging, functional MR imaging (which we are doing less of but we are acquiring resting state data), MR spectroscopy, and genetics. In DIAGNOSE we also use positron emission tomography (PET).

BACKGROUND

CTE is a neurodegenerative disease characterized by the deposition of hyperphosphorylated tau in neurons and astrocytes in a pattern that is unique when compared to other tauopathies (Chapter 2).[1,2] CTE is characterized by focal perivascular neurofibrillary tangles primarily at the depths of the cerebral sulci, and it spreads throughout the brain from there. It is not characterized by β-amyloid plaques as seen in Alzheimer's disease (AD). Supporting this last point, we now have tau and florbetapir amyloid imaging in 20 former NFL players, 4 Alzheimer's subjects, and 6 controls; not one of the

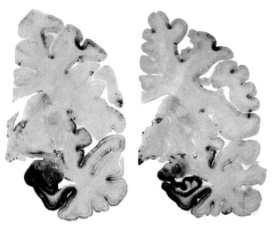

FIG. 11.1 Postmortem tau distribution in two professional football players. (With permission from McKee AC, Cantu RC, Nowinski CJ, et al. Chronic traumatic encephalopathy in athletes: progressive tauopathy after repetitive head injury. *Journal of Neuropathology and Experimental Neurology.* 2009;68(7):709–735.)

former NFL players with presumed CTE was positive for florbetapir, which is really telling. Of further note, CTE is most often diagnosed in former professional athletes in such sports as boxing and football when players are exposed to repetitive head impacts resulting in concussion and subconcussive trauma. Evidence indicates that a history of repetitive head trauma is necessary but not sufficient for the development of CTE (e.g., Refs. 3–5).

Fig. 11.1 shows the postmortem deposition of tau in the depths of the sulci and the medial temporal lobes in two former professional football players. One of the areas that we are starting to focus on is obtaining imaging measures in the area of these deep sulci. We have a computer scientist in our laboratory who is able to image much closer than 1 mm, and with such high resolution imaging we may be able to use MRI to map the structure onto what we see in postmortem images. We also know from the animal work of Dr. Lee Goldstein (Chapter 5) that blast injuries and impact injuries look very similar to one another pathologically.[6]

IN VIVO BRAIN IMAGING FINDINGS IN FORMER NFL PLAYERS
Cortical Atrophy and Cavum Septum Pellucidum

What about brain injury findings in these former NFL players? Brain atrophy has been found at postmortem by Dr. Ann McKee (Chapter 2),[1,2] and we also see it on MRI. Generally, it is regional atrophy that one sees in these NFL players on MR images. This is likely linked to repetitive head trauma or possibly CTE. One can see the atrophy in Fig. 11.2 in this NFL player both frontally and in the temporal lobe, even just looking at the whole brain against the skull.

We also heard earlier about the CSP, which, for the most part, closes at birth. In a small number of normal individuals it doesn't close right away but instead closes later or not at all. It is also seen in patients with schizophrenia. So when we talk about biomarkers, we need to realize that biomarkers may not be specific to one disease, but when you take into account the total constellation of biomarkers, that tells one something about a pattern of disease, further underscoring the fact that an individual biomarker doesn't have to be specific to one disorder. We certainly see CSP at postmortem in CTE (Fig. 11.3), and we also see it in the MRI scans of symptomatic retired NFL players as well (Fig. 11.3).[7] In fact, there is increasing frequency of CSP in the worse neuropathological stages.[2]

Fig. 11.4 shows a boxer with CSP, and here it is not only fenestrated with holes but also completely obliterated at the posterior end. This type of fenestrated CSP results from impacts to the head. Does it happen in every boxer? No, of course not. Does it happen more than you would expect in the general public? Yes.[8,9]

We assessed CSP in 72 former NFL players and 14 controls from the DETECT study. The NFL players had a higher rate of CSP, a greater length of CSP, and a greater ratio of CSP length to septum length (Fig. 11.5).[7] Furthermore, in the NFL group there was a greater length of CSP that was significantly associated with decreased performance on a list learning task (NAB List A Immediate Recall) and decreased test scores on a measure estimated verbal intelligence (Wide Range Achievement Test, Version 4 [WRAT-4]).

Volumes of Hippocampus, Amygdala, Cingulate Gyrus, and Thalamus

Another area that we investigated is volume of the hippocampus, the amygdala, and the cingulate gyrus, all areas that have been thought to be important in repetitive brain trauma (Fig. 11.6). This study comprised 86 symptomatic former NFL players and 22 controls from the DETECT study. Relative to the controls, the players had a significantly reduced volume in the left and right amygdala, hippocampus, and cingulate gyrus. The players also demonstrated worse mood and behavior, as well as reduced verbal memory. Within the NFL group, the reduced volume of the left and right cingulate gyrus was associated with worse attention and psychomotor

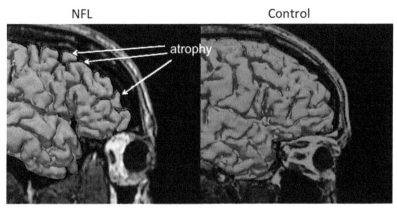

FIG. 11.2 Cortical atrophy in a former National Football League (NFL) football player compared with a control individual. (Figure courtesy of Dr. Martha Shenton.)

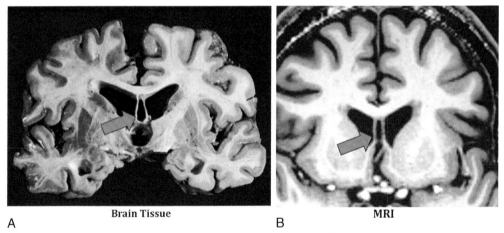

FIG. 11.3 Cavum septum pellucidum. (**A**) Gross pathology; (**B**) MRI. (Gross pathology image courtesy of Dr. Ann McKee. MRI image courtesy of Dr. Martha Shenton.)

speed. Additionally, reduced volume of the right hippocampus was associated with impaired visual memory (Lepage et al., unpublished data).

The other area we looked at was the thalamus (Fig. 11.7), which is a kind of way station in the brain, and here again we evaluated 86 symptomatic former NFL players from the DETECT study. We measured the right and left thalamic volume, which was negatively associated with total years of playing football, and right thalamic volume, which was also associated with the age of the first exposure in football even when adjusting for total years of play. Thus the younger the age one started playing football the greater the volume loss, even though we are talking about NFL players who are now retired—that is an important point because the former NFL players

studied are now in their late 40s into their 60s. We also found that the reduced volume of the left thalamus was associated with worse visual memory, whereas the larger volume of the right hippocampus was associated with worse mood and behavioral symptoms (Schultz et al., unpublished data). Thus there seems to be a definite risk involved with starting to play football earlier. The total number of years of play is associated with reduced volume but not nearly to the extent as is age of starting to play. This is a very important take-home message.

Basic Principles of Diffusion Tensor Imaging

We next provide a brief tutorial on diffusion imaging.

In diffusion imaging, we are talking about how water diffuses in the brain. If one were to drop ink on a tissue, it will disperse in all directions equally—producing a circle of ink as it spreads out—and this is referred to as isotropic diffusion (Fig. 11.8). If, on the other hand, one were to drop ink on a newspaper, it will disperse less in all directions than is the case for tissue, and this is due to the fibers in the newspaper that restrict the spread of the ink, producing an ellipsoid shape instead of a circle—and this is referred to as anisotropic diffusion (Fig. 11.8). This can be seen in the brain, where water diffuses more equally in all directions in gray matter and is isotropic, whereas water diffuses in a more restricted fashion in white matter, along the direction of the myelinated axons, and is anisotropic (Fig. 11.9). Thus, by using diffusion tensor imaging we can take advantage of the directionality of water in order to analyze the microstructural characteristics of brain tissue, which is very much affected in traumatic brain injury.

Repetitive Head Trauma and Possible Effects of Age at First Exposure to Trauma

One of the studies we performed in former NFL players was to look at the age of onset when someone begins to play. This study was conducted by Julie Stamm, as part of her PhD dissertation with Dr. Stern, Dr. Martha Shenton, and Dr. Inga Koerte. In this study, published in the *Journal of Neurotrauma*, we looked at how age of the first exposure to football might alter the structure of the corpus callosum white matter tracts. We chose to examine the corpus callosum with diffusion imaging because the corpus callosum is the largest white matter tract in the brain and when there is an impact to the head, the corpus callosum may be stretched along with the rest of the brain. It is important to point out that between the ages of 9 and 12 seems to be a critical time period for brain development of white matter and myelination.[10]

In this study, there were 42 former NFL players between the ages of 40 and 69 from the DETECT sample. We divided them into two groups based on their age of first exposure to tackle football, under age 12 or age 12 and older. We then matched them for their

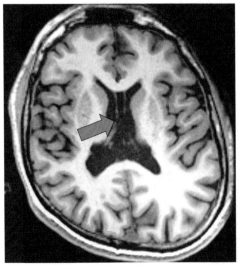

FIG. 11.4 MRI of a cavum septum pellucidum that has been fenestrated, particularly in its posterior extent. (Figure courtesy of Dr. Martha Shenton.)

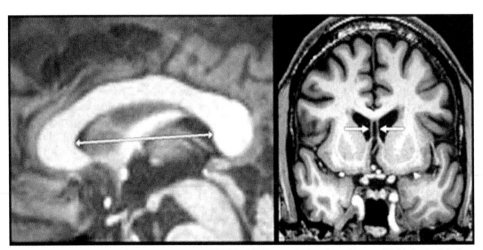

FIG. 11.5 MRI measures of cavum septi pellucidi. (With permission from Koerte IK, Hufschmidt J, Muehlmann M, et al. Cavum septi pellucidi in symptomatic former professional football players. *Journal of Neurotrauma*. 2016;33(4):346–353.)

current, chronological age and analyzed the corpus callosum with diffusion tensor imaging. We divided the corpus callosum into five subregions. Fig. 11.10 is an example of the kind of information one can see when

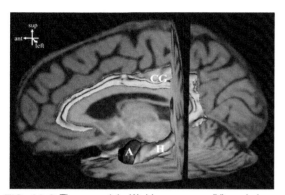

FIG. 11.6 The amygdala (A), hippocampus (H), and cingulate gyrus (CG) are important structures in understanding repetitive brain trauma. (Figure courtesy of Drs. Martha Shenton and Inga Koerte.)

extracting fiber tracts that comprise five subregions of the corpus callosum.

We found that those who started playing football before the age of 12 had lower fractional anisotropy—which means that the directionality of diffusion was decreased, meaning there was less white matter integrity in the anterior three regions of the corpus callosum. This finding suggests that white matter microstructural integrity is abnormal. There was also higher radial diffusivity—a measure of myelin integrity (higher is worse)—suggesting reduced diameter of myelin sheath or loss of myelination. So in summary, we see altered microstructural integrity of the anterior corpus callosum in former NFL players who began tackle football before age 12 compared with those who were 12 and older when they began to play tack football.[11] We think that the anterior corpus callosum neuroanatomy, combined with incomplete and rapid myelination between the ages of 8 to 12, may predispose the anterior corpus callosum to detrimental effects of repetitive head

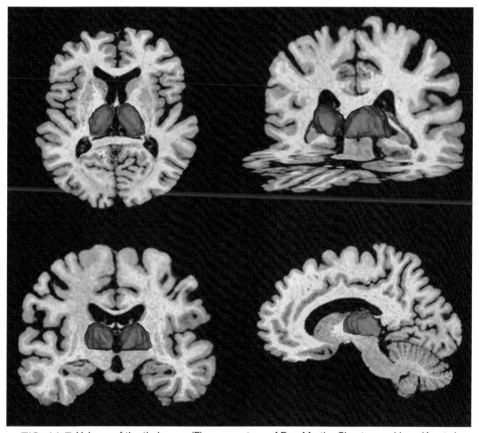

FIG. 11.7 Volume of the thalamus. (Figure courtesy of Drs. Martha Shenton and Inga Koerte.)

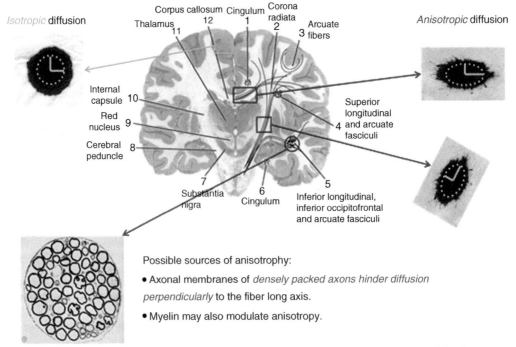

Possible sources of anisotrophy:

• Axonal membranes of *densely packed axons hinder diffusion*
perpendicularly to the fiber long axis.

• Myelin may also modulate anisotropy.

FIG. 11.8 Water diffusion in the brain has directionality. (Courtesy of Drs. Sylvain Bouix and Gordon Kindlmann.)

impact experienced during this critical period of neurodevelopment.

We should note limitations of this study, which include the fact that we were investigating a unique cohort of symptomatic former NFL players who are middle age; we do not know what the results would look like in those who only played through high school or college. We were also not able to take into account whether the findings would be equally true for children starting to play football today, as the game is played differently now compared to 30 years ago. Lastly, we note that our imaging findings do not necessarily indicate that a former NFL player has or will develop CTE. We do think, however, that our imaging findings are one of a number of factors that may increase the probability of developing CTE at some point in time. It is our hope that if we can detect imaging abnormalities during life, then we can better understand risk factors for CTE. In the future, combining imaging risks factors with genetic and other risk factors may allow us to estimate individuals' risk for developing CTE if they choose to play football. Right now we know that the risk of developing CTE is higher if you play football, but we also know that not everyone who plays football ends up with CTE.

BRAIN IMAGING FINDINGS IN VIVO IN PROFESSIONAL SOCCER PLAYERS

The next group that we looked at is professional soccer players. We wanted to examine repetitive, subconcussive head impacts. We focused on former professional soccer players in Germany who've had repetitive subconcussive blows to the head. Dr. Koerte conducted this research with colleagues from Germany and with members of Dr. Shenton's laboratory. We compared active elite soccer players with competitive swimmers. We included only those with subconcussive blows to the head. The split in the data between these two groups was so large that it is something I've not often seen in my prior research. There was a complete separation between groups, with soccer players showing abnormally increased radial diffusivity, suggesting reduced myelination compared to the swimmers.[12] This was the first study to investigate subconcussive blows to the head using MR imaging.

In another study, we included former professional soccer players. And here we included those with and without concussion, although we highlighted those who stated they had a concussion sometime during their lifetime. We found that there was pronounced cortical thinning with age in the former professional

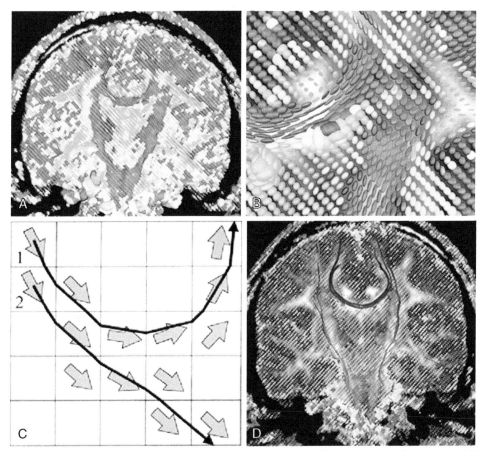

FIG. 11.9 Diffusion tensor imaging. (**A and B**) At each location the diffusion behavior of water is modeled as an ellipsoid. In medical imaging this ellipsoid is called a diffusion tensor. (**C**) The major diffusion direction is associated with the tangent to a curve. (**D**) The curve is estimated from its tangents to form tracts. (Figure courtesy of Dr. Martha Shenton.)

soccer players compared with controls, whose cortical thicknesses only slightly decreased with age[13] (Fig. 11.11). Note in Fig. 11.11 that the triangles are the goalkeepers who don't use their head as much, and the circles are the soccer players who had past concussions.

REPETITIVE HEAD IMPACTS IN UNIVERSITY HOCKEY PLAYERS

We also looked at university ice hockey players from Canada, and here we compared pre- and postseason evaluation. Postseason scans showed a higher mean diffusivity—a measure that may indicate more space between axons. There were three participants who suffered from concussion during the season who are shown in red in Fig. 11.12. Interestingly two were much

worse postseason but there is one who doesn't look any different from those who did not experience a concussion[14] (Fig. 11.12). In a similar study on college football players, we followed up on the players 6 months after the end of the play season and our results indicate that these abnormalities may return to normal after a period of no contact rest (Mayinger et al., unpublished data).

ADVANCED IMAGING MEASURES FOR USE IN THE DIAGNOSE U01 GRANT

Introduction

Some important questions are what do these findings really mean and how reversible are they? It seems obvious that over time if you keep having repetitive hits to the head causing changes in the brain, it's probably

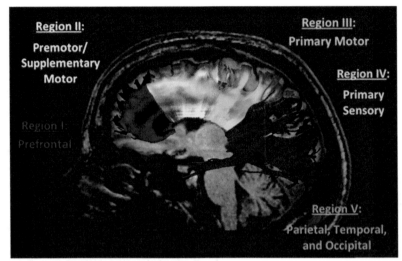

FIG. 11.10 Corpus callosum divided into five brain regions. (From Stamm JM, Koerte IK, Muehlmann M, et al. Age at first exposure to football is associated with altered corpus callosum white matter microstructure in former professional football players. *Journal of Neurotrauma*. 2015;32(22):1768–1776.)

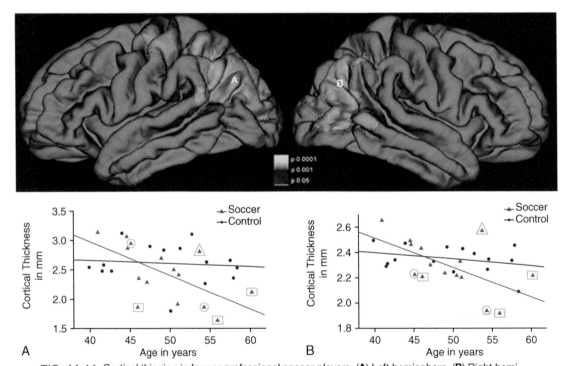

FIG. 11.11 Cortical thinning in former professional soccer players. (**A**) Left hemisphere. (**B**) Right hemisphere. *Triangle*, goal keeper; *circles*, past TBI; *squares*, highest lifetime headers. (With permission from Koerte IK, Mayinger M, Muehlmann M, et al. Cortical thinning in former professional soccer players. *Brain Imaging and Behavior*. 2015. http://dx.doi.org/10.1007/s11682-015-9442-0.)

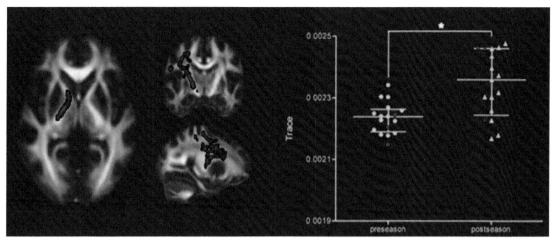

FIG. 11.12 Higher mean diffusivity in ice hockey players post- versus preseason. Left panel shows areas of the brain that changed between pre- and postseason. Right panel shows mean diffusivity. Participants who suffered from concussion during the season are shown in red. (With permission from Koerte IK, Kaufmann D, Hartl E, et al. A prospective study of physician-observed concussion during a varsity university hockey season: white matter integrity in ice hockey players. Part 3 of 4. *Neurosurgical Focus*. 2012;33(6):E3: 1–7.)

not good for you. But what kind of rest period do you need? What kind of guidelines should we have for children? What is the right age for children to safely start football? Although there are medications to treat some of the symptoms of CTE, as discussed by Dr. Andrew Budson (Chapter 9), can we identify targets for medications to slow or even prevent the disease itself? These are all questions that really need to be addressed. We are working toward finding answers to these questions with our new U01 grant.

In this new research project, DIAGNOSE CTE, we will be evaluating 120 former NFL players, 60 former college players, and 60 no-contact sport athletes as a control group. These individuals will undergo a number of different measures now and in the follow-up 3 years later. The main goals are:
- To examine the incidence and prevalence of presumed CTE.
- To treat and prevent long-term consequences of repetitive impacts, including CTE.
- To detect changes early (prior to brain degeneration and possibly even prior to symptoms) and to set the stage to intervene with disease-modifying or neuroprotective compounds when they become available.
- To determine specific risk factors for CTE and other long-term consequences of repetitive head impacts so that appropriate recommendations can be made to reduce later life problems.

PET Imaging Using β-Amyloid and Tau Ligands

I would like to mention that we will be using PET imaging to look at both β-amyloid and tau. We expect to see both tau and β-amyloid deposition in patients with AD. We predict that we will see tau deposition but no β-amyloid deposition in patients at risk for CTE, whereas in controls we predict that we will see neither β-amyloid nor tau deposition. This part of the new U01 is headed by Dr. Eric Reiman.

Free-Water Imaging

Another technique we plan to use is free-water imaging. It is based on the work that we've done in schizophrenia. A computer scientist in our group took what we discussed previously regarding isotropic diffusion, and he separated the MRI signal into two parts: one due to extracellular or free water, which we think of as edema or neuroinflammation, and the other due to water surrounding or within brain tissue, which we think of as intracellular. Although because of the resolution we cannot truly say intracellular, we instead refer to the water in the brain tissue compartment. We think, however, that this intracellular water reflects neurodegeneration. We have used this technique to image brain tumors such as meningiomas.[15,16] We have also used it to investigate free water and water in the brain tissue compartment in first-episode schizophrenia and healthy controls.[17] In that study we found primarily extracellular water differences between the groups, suggesting widespread neuroinflammation in those with first-episode schizophrenia, but there was also a small amount of brain tissue compartment changes in frontal lobe areas, which suggests that neurodegenerative changes are already beginning to take place. By comparison, patients with chronic schizophrenia (living with the disorder for 15 years on average) have few extracellular water differences compared with controls, but the neurodegenerative changes in the brain tissue compartment are many.[18] What we want to do now is to apply this free-water technique to former NFL players and college players to investigate extracellular free water that might indicate early, possibly neuroinflammatory, changes in the brain and tissue compartment alterations that may indicate neurodegenerative changes in the brain. As Dr. Goldstein pointed out, neuroinflammation isn't necessarily a bad thing in and of itself; it may be protective initially, but at some point it becomes neurodegenerative and we don't know exactly when or why.

Subject-Specific Analyses: Precision Medicine Approach

Another area we want to investigate is subject-specific analyses. These analyses fit into what NIH calls a Precision Medicine Approach, and it gets back to what the clinician wants to know, similar to some of the images and case vignettes that Dr. Budson reviewed this morning (Chapter 9). After all, we are treating individual patients, so we don't want to only talk about groups. Accordingly, one of the computer scientists in our group has been working to develop a normative atlas in which a group of normal controls is matched with all variables except the ones that we think are the most important, such as having repetitive head impacts to the brain. He has completed one study investigating mild TBI in those who have experienced a single mild TBI (so they are not at all going to be in a CTE group) and who have persistent postconcussive symptoms. These individuals are clearly in the minority, as 80% of those who experience a concussion recover completely, with about 15% to 20% who experience persistent symptoms, even after one concussion. These individuals have been referred to as "the miserable minority."[19]

What we've done is to establish a way to assess each individual compared to a normative atlas.[20] Thus, we can look at someone who has had postconcussive symptoms for more than 5 years and actually find regional abnormalities that fit well with what we know

about their neuropsychological test performance. We now want to apply this method in the DIAGNOSE CTE project with the former NFL players, college players, and controls (Chapter 3).

Fig. 11.13 provides an example. The red lines represent 3.58 standard deviations above and below the mean for 178 areas in the brain divided into left gray matter, right gray matter, left white matter, and right white matter. If one looks at the normal control subjects, one can see there are two outliers. If one looks at the subjects with persistent postconcussive symptoms, however, one can see that almost every subject was in the borderline or abnormal range for one or more regions. What surprised us, however, was that the greatest alterations were in the gray matter, where we found primarily increases in fractional anisotropy, suggesting possible microgliosis.[20]

Beyond Diffusion Tensor Imaging

Another area we have focused on is to go beyond standard diffusion tensor imaging. One issue in standard diffusion tensor imaging is that where fibers cross one finds lower anisotropy, making it difficult to track these fibers through the brain. We solved this problem with the help of another computer scientist in our group, and we are now able to look at more than just isolated fiber tracts that stop because of crossing fibers.[21,22] Additionally, we can now see more fibers using multitensor tractography and even full-brain tractography (Fig. 11.14).

We can obtain this kind of information from anyone we put into the magnet. When done correctly, the imaging data from different brain regions correlates quite well with cognitive, behavioral, and emotional dysfunctions that are observed. Note, however, if research is conducted across multiple sites, harmonizing the data is needed, particularly for diffusion images which are more variable even when using the same make and model of the scanner in different locations.[23,24] We have developed a harmonization algorithm to address this issue.[23]

SUMMARY AND CONCLUSIONS

In summary, one of the goals of research in CTE is to develop imaging biomarkers that are associated with the postmortem findings in CTE and with the symptoms associated with presumed CTE. These imaging biomarkers can then serve as surrogate biomarkers of CTE with the hope that we can stage the disease in vivo when those at risk are still alive and when we can perhaps intervene as treatments become available.

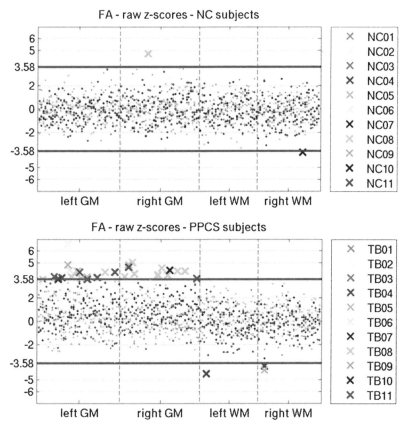

FIG. 11.13 Fractional anisotropy (FA) summary maps for populations. *GM*, gray matter; *NC*, normal control; *PPCS*, persistent postconcussive symptoms; *WM*, white matter. See text for additional details. (With permission from Bouix S, Pasternak O, Rathi Y, Pelavin PE, Zafonte R, Shenton ME. Increased gray matter diffusion anisotropy in patients with persistent post-concussive symptoms following mild traumatic brain injury. *PLoS One*. 2013;8(6):e66205.)

Specifically, we want to develop biomarkers of early changes in the brain prior to neurodegeneration and perhaps even prior to symptoms, if possible, thereby setting the stage to intervene with disease-modifying or neuroprotective compounds as they become available. Additionally, we want to determine specific imaging risk factors of CTE and other long-term consequences of repetitive impacts so that appropriate recommendations can be made to reduce later life problems. Finally, the words that need to be said over and over again are that repetitive head trauma is really the most important risk factor for CTE.

In closing, we note that we've come a long way. Some refer to imaging as the new phrenology. We,

however, would argue that one cannot have new discoveries without having the right tools. We have some of the right tools now, and we can link together brain-behavior relations in a manner that was heretofore not possible. We've thus come a long way from phrenology to the imaging of today. Thank you for your attention.

DISCLOSURE

Dr. Shenton receives grant support from the National Institutes of Health, the Veterans Administration, and the Department of Defense.

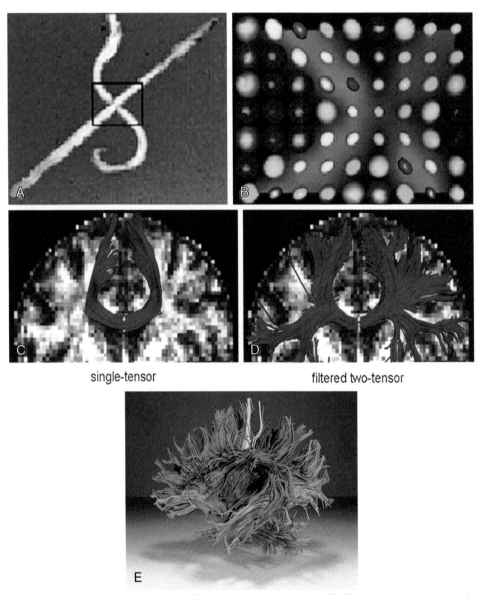

FIG. 11.14 Multitensor tractography. (**A**) Crossing white matter tracts. (**B**) Ellipsoids created by crossing white matter tracts. Note the isotropic (circular) ellipsoid where the tracts cross. (**C**) Single-tensor tractography. (**D**) Filtered two-tensor tractography. (**E**) Whole brain tractography. (Panels (**A**) to (**D**) from Malcolm JG, Shenton ME, Rathi Y. Neural tractography using an unscented Kalman filter. *Information Processing in Medical Imaging*. 2009;21:126–138. Panel (**E**) from O'Donnell, Banks, Kindlmann, and Westin, Laboratory of Mathematics in Imaging, and Kubicki and Shenton, Psychiatry Neuroimaging Laboratory, Harvard Medical School.)

REFERENCES

1. McKee AC, Cantu RC, Nowinski CJ, et al. Chronic traumatic encephalopathy in athletes: progressive tauopathy after repetitive head injury. *Journal of Neuropathology and Experimental Neurology.* 2009;68(7):709–735.

2. McKee AC, Stern RA, Nowinski CJ, et al. The spectrum of disease in chronic traumatic encephalopathy. *Brain.* 2013;136(Pt 1):43–64.

3. Baugh CM, Stamm JM, Riley DO, et al. Chronic traumatic encephalopathy: neurodegeneration following repetitive concussive and subconcussive brain trauma. *Brain Imaging and Behavior.* 2012;6(2):244–254.

4. Koerte IK, Lin AP, Willems A, et al. A review of neuroimaging findings in repetitive brain trauma. *Brain Pathology.* 2015;25(3):318–349.

5. McKee AC, Alosco ML, Huber BR. Repetitive head impacts and chronic traumatic encephalopathy. *Neurosurgery Clinics of North America.* 2016;27(4):529–535.

6. Goldstein LE, Fisher AM, Tagge CA, et al. Chronic traumatic encephalopathy in blast-exposed military veterans and a blast neurotrauma mouse model. *Science Translational Medicine.* 2012;4(134):134ra60.

7. Koerte IK, Hufschmidt J, Muehlmann M, et al. Cavum septi pellucidi in symptomatic former professional football players. *Journal of Neurotrauma.* 2016;33(4):346–353.

8. Orrison WW, Hanson EH, Alamo T, et al. Traumatic brain injury: a review and high-field MRI findings in 100 unarmed combatants using a literature-based checklist approach. *Journal of Neurotrauma.* 2009;26(5):689–701.

9. Smith DH, Johnson VE, Stewart W. Chronic neuropathologies of single and repetitive TBI: substrates of dementia? *Nature Reviews Neurology.* 2013;9(4):211–221.

10. Lebel C, Beaulieu C. Longitudinal development of human brain wiring continues from childhood into adulthood. *Journal of Neuroscience.* 2011;31(30):10937–10947.

11. Stamm JM, Koerte IK, Muehlmann M, et al. Age at first exposure to football is associated with altered corpus callosum white matter microstructure in former professional football players. *Journal of Neurotrauma.* 2015;32(22):1768–1776.

12. Koerte IK, Ertl-Wagner B, Reiser M, Zafonte R, Shenton ME. White matter integrity in the brains of professional soccer players without a symptomatic concussion. *JAMA.* 2012;308(18):1859–1861.

13. Koerte IK, Mayinger M, Muehlmann M, et al. Cortical thinning in former professional soccer players. *Brain Imaging and Behavior.* 2016;10(3):792–798.

14. Koerte IK, Kaufmann D, Hartl E, et al. A prospective study of physician-observed concussion during a varsity university hockey season: white matter integrity in ice hockey players. Part 3 of 4. *Neurosurgical Focus.* 2012;33(6). E3: 1–7.

15. Pasternak O, Assaf Y. Evaluation of tissue condition within cerebral edema by free water elimination. In: *Proceedings of the 15th meeting of the Organization for Human Brain Mapping (HBM); 2009; San Francisco, CA*; 2009.

16. Pasternak O, Sochen N, Gur Y, Intrator N, Assaf Y. Free water elimination and mapping from diffusion MRI. *Magnetic Resonance in Medicine.* 2009;62(3):717–730.

17. Pasternak O, Westin CF, Bouix S, et al. Excessive extracellular volume reveals a neurodegenerative pattern in schizophrenia onset. *Journal of Neuroscience.* 2012;32(48):17365–17372.

18. Pasternak O, Kubicki M, Shenton ME. In vivo imaging of neuroinflammation in schizophrenia. *Schizophrenia Research.* 2016;173(3):200–212.

19. Ruff RM, Camenzuli L, Mueller J. Miserable minority: emotional risk factors that influence the outcome of a mild traumatic brain injury. *Brain Injury.* 1996;10(8):551–565.

20. Bouix S, Pasternak O, Rathi Y, Pelavin PE, Zafonte R, Shenton ME. Increased gray matter diffusion anisotropy in patients with persistent post-concussive symptoms following mild traumatic brain injury. *PLoS One.* 2013;8(6):e66205.

21. Malcolm JG, Shenton ME, Rathi Y. Neural tractography using an unscented Kalman filter. *Information Processing in Medical Imaging.* 2009;21:126–138.

22. Rathi Y, Kubicki M, Bouix S, et al. Statistical analysis of fiber bundles using multi-tensor tractography: application to first-episode schizophrenia. *Magnetic Resonance Imaging.* 2011;29(4):507–515.

23. Mirzaalian H, de Pierrefeu A, Savadjiev P, et al. Harmonizing diffusion MRI data across multiple sites and scanners. *Medical Image Computing and Computer-Assisted Intervention.* 2015;9349:12–19.

24. Mirzaalian H, Ning L, Savadjiev P, et al. Inter-site and inter-scanner diffusion MRI data harmonization. *NeuroImage.* 2016;135:311–323.

CHAPTER 12

From Chronic Traumatic Encephalopathy Biomarkers to Therapeutics: What We Need to Know to Design Clinical Trials

RAMON DIAZ-ARRASTIA • FRANCK AMYOT • MARGALIT HABER • CAROL MOORE • KIMBRA KENNEY

INTRODUCTION

Thank you so much for inviting me to this terrific symposium. It's really great to be here in the hub of chronic traumatic encephalopathy (CTE). I don't work on CTE—I work mainly in emergency rooms and with hospital-based patients with traumatic brain injury (TBI), but I have been following the impressive work of Dr. Ann McKee, Dr. Robert Stern, Dr. Lee Goldstein, and many others in this group over the years. When I was asked to give a talk on biomarkers and therapeutics of CTE, I first thought, "this is going to be a short talk," since the field is very much in its infancy. Then I thought a little bit more about it, and I put a twist in the title, "what do we need to know in order to design clinical trials," because I do think we are on the cusp of starting to do clinical trials with individuals who have presumed CTE. I don't think we need to understand everything about CTE from pathology to pathophysiology, preclinical models, and signs and symptoms to start clinical trials, but the more we understand, the better. In fact, that understanding is best when the basic studies proceed in an iterative fashion with therapeutic development. We learned from other fields that as we go forward in clinical trials, we also go back and inform our preclinical models with what the clinical trials taught us, and we can look at lessons from pathology as well. So learning these lessons in relation to CTE is the task that I gave to myself.

TERMINOLOGY

Endophenotypes

In order to conduct the next generation of clinical trials in TBI, and the first generation of clinical trials in CTE,

we are going to have to understand endophenotypes. An endophenotype is an internal or intermediate phenotype that is closer to the underlying pathophysiology of the disease, whether it is genetic or environmental. By definition, an endophenotype must be a continuous, quantitative variable—as opposed to a phenotype, which is usually a categorical variable (e.g., yes or no; the patient has the disease or they don't). An endophenotype can be measured quantitatively through physiological, biochemical, or imaging—and eventually pathological—techniques.[1] For any one phenotype there are potentially many endophenotypes that contribute to the expression of that ultimate phenotype, with different endophenotypes sometimes contributing in different ways in different patients. Synonyms for endophenotype include endotype and subphenotype.

For example, we know that for the syndrome of coronary artery disease there are potentially multiple endophenotypes that contribute to how that phenotype develops, such as hypertension, hyperlipidemia, vascular inflammation, and potentially many others. When a cardiologist works with patients who have coronary heart disease, he doesn't just give them a drug for coronary heart disease; he measures their blood pressure, their cholesterol, and their C-reactive protein, and the therapy chosen is targeted at the set of endophenotypes that are active in particular patients. I believe that it will be similar for conditions such as CTE—therapy will need to be directed at the endophenotype rather than the phenotype. Phenotypes are necessarily going to be heterogeneous based on the underlying endophenotype differences.

So what are the endophenotypes of TBI? We don't necessarily know them all, but we know that the major

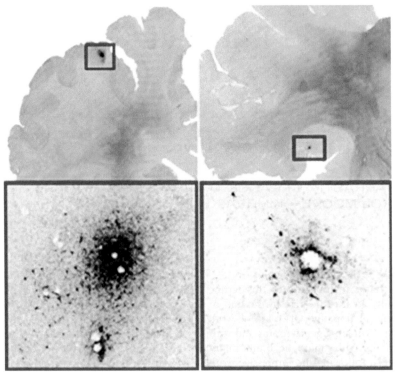

FIG. 12.1 Perivascular deposits in chronic traumatic encephalopathy. (Figure courtesy of Dr. Ann McKee and Dr. Daniel Perl.)

ones are likely to include inflammation, diffuse axonal injury, and diffuse vascular injury. I am going to focus mostly on diffuse vascular injury. We heard from the talks of Dr. McKee (Chapter 2) and Dr. Thor Stein (Chapter 8) how vascular injury is a very prominent feature of CTE (Fig. 12.1). There are, of course, other endophenotypes of CTE, such as a tauopathy endophenotype.

Biomarkers

The other thing that I wanted to discuss—and we heard about this topic from Dr. Kaj Blennow (Chapter 10)—is that biomarkers are going to be the way in which we measure these endophenotypes. Biomarkers have many uses. Here is a nosology of biomarkers that was arrived at by consensus conference between the National Institutes of Health (NIH) and the Food and Drug Administration (FDA)[2] (Box 12.1).

Diagnostic biomarkers are going to be important in clinical medicine and will be critically important for the development of therapeutics. We also need to have prognostic biomarkers to categorize patients by the likelihood of disease progression. So the question

becomes not just, "did the patient have a TBI or not?" but is instead, "is this a brain injury that is likely to progress over time and become a neurodegenerative disease such as CTE?" Predictive biomarkers categorize patients by the likelihood of their response to a particular treatment. For example, if we had a biomarker of inflammation that could potentially be a predictive biomarker for a patient who is likely to respond to an antiinflammatory therapy. Pharmacodynamic biomarkers are dynamic and can show the biological response to a particular therapy because, as we know, patients differ in the dose they require, and we need a pharmacodynamic biomarker to determine the correct dose to treat a particular patient and see the response.

Types of Studies

We need biomarkers to measure endophenotypes that can be aligned with and developed iteratively between clinical and preclinical studies. We will need to start with observational studies in humans, where we can assess the natural history of endophenotypes in patients with TBI and identify a subset of individuals who are likely to develop long-term problems and therefore likely to merit if we give therapy. Once we are at that point with observational studies in humans, we are going to have to go back to the animal models and work with folks like Dr. Goldstein (Chapter 5) and many others in the room to confirm in a preclinical model the mechanistic benefit of therapy. We will need to establish the pharmacodynamic relevance of those biomarkers for that treatment in the animal models. Only once we do those things, then will we be ready to do biomarker-driven phase II clinical trials in humans, which can establish the optimal dose, timing, and duration of therapy. So what I am going to tell you now for the rest of my time today is our results from particular phase II clinical trial in humans we recently completed in Bethesda, Maryland.

MICROVASCULAR INJURY

The particular phase IIA clinical trial we conducted focused on microvascular injuries as endophenotype because we have many drugs that are widely used in clinical medicine approved by the FDA and the European Medicines Agency that are active on the vasculature. Vascular biology is a very mature area of science,

and we can certainly benefit from what our colleagues in that area of medicine have learned. We know that sildenafil—the drug that I am going to tell you most about—has potent effects on the vasculature of the brain and the body. But that is not the only one. HMG-CoA reductase inhibitors, such as statins, have very potent effects on endothelial biology, in promoting vascular health, are antiinflammatory, and are proangiogenic. Erythropoietin has been tried and failed in clinical trials of very severe TBI. There are many others, including omega-3 fatty acids, granulocyte-macrophage colony-stimulating factor, bone-marrow derived stem cells, and there are also nonpharmacological approaches such as aerobic exercise.

Cerebral Microcirculation and the Neurovascular Unit

Fig. 12.2A summarizes the anatomy of the cerebral microvasculature,[3] and Fig. 12.2B shows the actual anatomy from a vascular corrosion cast.[4] Blood to the cortex is supplied by this rich capillary bed that comes off of these pial arterial vessels at right angles to them, penetrating through the pia. Because of the anatomy of these blood vessels, they are very susceptible to the shearing, stretching, and mechanical forces that result from TBI, whether it is severe TBI, mild TBI, or concussion.

Diffuse Vascular Injury After TBI

We've known for a long time that diffuse vascular injury is very common and nearly universal in lethal TBI. Fig. 12.3 shows an example from pathology, showing diffuse vascular injury in the penetrating blood vessels.[5] We have recognized more recently that diffuse vascular injury is not only a feature in severe TBI but also in mild TBI.

Fig. 12.4 is from a study that was conducted by our colleague at the National Institute of Neurological Disorders and Stroke, Dr. Larry Latour, using MRI in people who present in emergency rooms with acute TBI. It shows the brain of a young woman involved in an automobile accident. She fell asleep at the wheel and ran off the road. She didn't hit anything, but she turned over her car as she was going over the side of the road. She may have had loss of consciousness, but if so it was very brief. She was found by witnesses outside of the car; she was conscious and knew what was going on and she was taken to an emergency room. She had a CT scan that was normal and was told she was very lucky and that she did not have a TBI. Fortunately, she enrolled in this study in which they performed an MRI, which included susceptibility sequences, and found

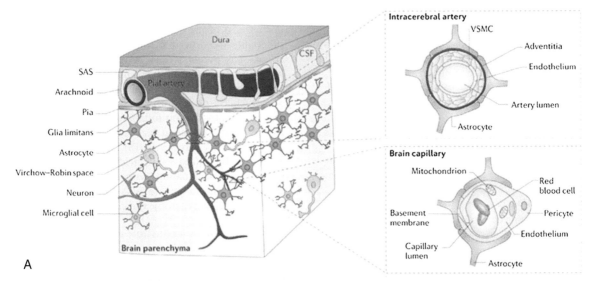

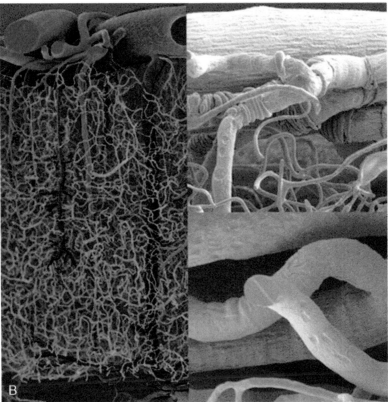

FIG. 12.2 Cerebral microcirculation and the neurovascular unit. **(A)** Diagram of the cerebral microcirculation and the neurovascular unit. **(B)** Example of that actual anatomy of the cerebral microcirculation from a vascular corrosion cast. ((A) From Zlokovic BV. Neurovascular pathways to neurodegeneration in Alzheimer's disease and other disorders. *Nature Reviews. Neuroscience*. November 3, 2011;12(12):723–738. http://dx.doi.org/10.1038/nrn3114. **(B)** From Weber B, Keller AL, Reichold J, Logothetis NK. The microvascular system of the striate and extrastriate visual cortex of the macaque. *Cerebral Cortex*. October 2008;18(10):2318–2330. http://dx.doi.org/10.1093/cercor/bhm259.)

these linear microhemorrhages, which are evidence of vascular injury in the deep vessels, at least one of which is associated with abnormal diffusion-weighted imaging indicating tissue damage.

Now, it is very rare to do an MRI at such an early period after a TBI, but it was done in this study and abnormalities similar to that of the young woman were found in approximately 25% of people who went to the emergency room and were diagnosed with a mild TBI with a negative CT scan. So these types of abnormal findings are not at all uncommon. The TRACK-TBI (Transforming Research and Clinical Knowledge in Traumatic

Brain Injury) Consortium has tracked such abnormalities as well. So this type of abnormality is a very common finding, and just because we don't see it on CT then it doesn't mean it is not there. The MRI is more sensitive than the CT scan, and note that this is a standard MRI that does not require diffusion tensor imaging.

Response of Cerebral Microvasculature to TBI

We've known about the damage from TBI to cerebral microvasculature for some time from animal models. Fig. 12.5 is from a study done at the University of Pennsylvania in which a primate was sacrificed 20 min after a TBI.[6] I want to point out the changes to endothelia after a brain injury. Here you can see the vesicles that are popping out of the endothelial wall—these are likely the exosomes that Dr. Stern (Chapter 3) and Dr. Blennow (Chapter 10) told you about.

Fig. 12.6 shows changes that can occur in the cerebral microvasculature after a TBI. These examples use the vascular corrosion cast technique. Panel A shows the normal precapillary arterial, and you can see that the endothelium is normally very smooth. Panel B shows the same vessels in a patient who died several days after a severe a TBI. You can see how the endothelial wall is thickened with abnormal folds and pits.[7,8]

In Vivo Imaging of Cerebral Microvasculature in Response to TBI

So how can we assess microvascular injury in humans? One way is to use dynamic contrast-enhanced MRI to assess blood-brain barrier dysfunction after TBI.

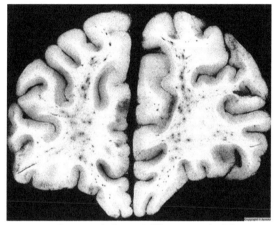

FIG. 12.3 Gross pathology of diffuse vascular injury after traumatic brain injury. (With permission from Graham DI, Lantos PL, eds. *Greenfield's Neuropathology*, 7th ed. London: Arnold; 2002.)

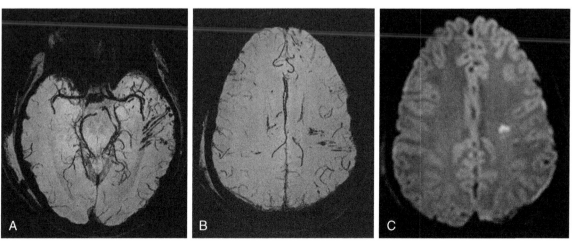

FIG. 12.4 MRI of diffuse vascular injury after mild traumatic brain injury. **(A and B)** Note linear microhemorrhages on susceptibility sequences. **(C)** Abnormal diffusion-weighted imaging indicating tissue damage. See text for additional details. (Figure courtesy of Larry Latour, PhD, NINDS/CNRM.)

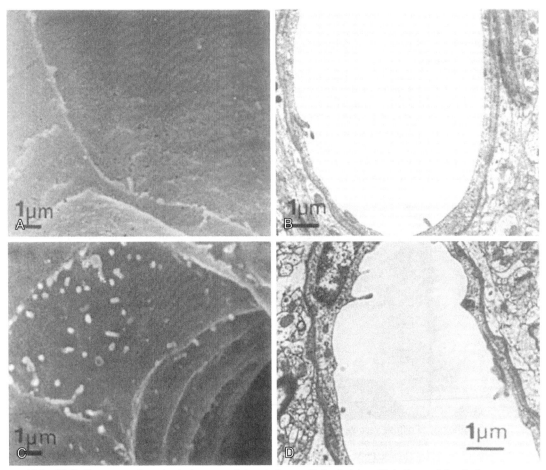

FIG. 12.5 Response of cerebral microvasculature to traumatic brain injury. Note the vesicles that are coming off of the endothelial wall in response to brain injury. **(A and B)** Control condition. **(C and D)** 20 min after TBI. (With permission from Maxwell WL, Irvine A, Adams JH, Graham DI, Gennarelli TA. Response of cerebral microvasculature to brain injury. *The Journal of Pathology*. August 1988;155(4):327–335.)

When you administer a bolus of gadolinium, there is a rapid shortening of the T1 signals, but in the intact blood-brain barrier the gadolinium stays within the blood vessel, and then that shortening dissipates very quickly and no signal is seen on MRI. On the other hand, when patients have some degree of blood-brain barrier dysfunction, some of the gadolinium enters the tissue and then washes out slowly, so the signal can be seen on MRI. Fig. 12.7 shows the use of this technique in amateur football players, in a study published recently by our colleague Dr. Alon Friedman. There is evidence of subtle blood-brain barrier dysfunction, even though in many cases these scans were acquired weeks and months after playing and not associated with particular concussions.

PHASE II STUDY: SILDENAFIL FOR CEREBROVASCULAR DYSFUNCTION IN CHRONIC TRAUMATIC BRAIN INJURY

So for the rest of my time I am going to tell you about the results of this recently completed phase II study, Sildenafil for Cerebrovascular Dysfunction in Chronic Traumatic Brain Injury. We wanted a potential therapy for cerebrovascular dysfunction after TBI, and the drug we used was sildenafil, better known from its brand name, Viagra.

Mechanism of Sildenafil

Sildenafil is a potent and highly specific phosphodiesterase (PDE) 5 inhibitor approved by the FDA for the treatment of erectile dysfunction and also for primary

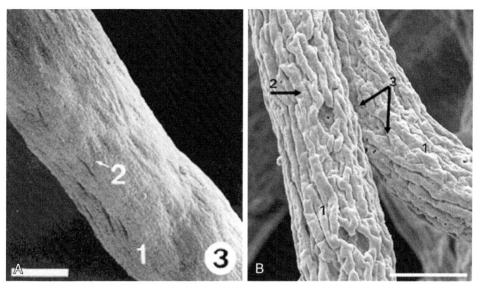

FIG. 12.6 Changes in cerebral microvasculature after a traumatic brain injury using the vascular corrosion cast technique. **(A)** Normal precapillary arteriole. Note that the endothelium is very smooth. **(B)** Precapillary arteriole in a patient who died several days after a severe a TBI. Note how the endothelial wall is thickened with abnormal folding and aggregations. Numbers identify cell nuclei. (**(A)** From Rodriguez-Baeza A, Reina-De La Torre F, Ortega-Sanchez M, Sahuquillo-Barris J. Perivascular structures in corrosion casts of the human central nervous system: a confocal laser and scanning electron microscope study. *The Anatomical Record*. October 1998;252(2):176–184. **(B)** From Rodríguez-Baeza A, Reina-de la Torre F, Poca A, Martí M, Garnacho A. Morphological features in human cortical brain microvessels after head injury: a three-dimensional and immunocytochemical study. *The Anatomical Record. Part A, Discoveries in Molecular, Cellular, and Evolutionary Biology*. July 2003;273(1):583–593.)

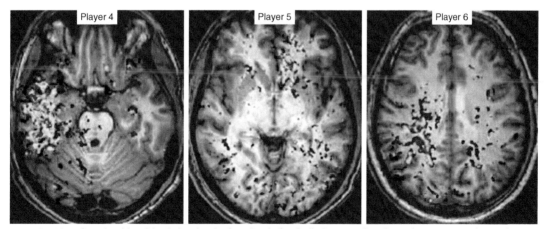

FIG. 12.7 Imaging blood-brain barrier dysfunction in football players using dynamic contrast-enhanced MRI. (With permission from Weissberg I, Veksler R, Kamintsky L, et al. Imaging blood-brain barrier dysfunction in football players. *JAMA Neurology*. November 2014;71(11):1453–1455. http://dx.doi.org/10.1001/jamaneurol.2014.2682.)

pulmonary hypertension. It potentiates nitric oxide sig-naling in the blood vessels, and it has been known in animal models of stroke to have neuroprotective and proangiogenic effects.[9]

When the endothelial cell senses that there is increased demand for blood flow, it activates nitric oxide synthetase that produces nitric oxide, which is a gas that diffuses to the smooth muscle cells and acti-vates guanylyl cyclase, which catalyzes the transforma-tion of GTP to cyclic GMP (cGMP), which then activates a number of other proteins that produces vasodilation. The cGMP signal is turned off by PDE 5, so sildenafil inhibits the hydrolysis of cGMP, thereby prolonging the nitric oxide signal. So patients with vascular dysfunc-tion from either diabetes or old age or whatever reason can often benefit by using these drugs.

Design of the Phase II Study

There were three groups in our study. The experimental group consisted of 24 patients with persistent TBI post-concussive symptoms for at least 6 months. They were studied with MRI using hypercapnia BOLD at base-line, before and after a single dose of sildenafil (50 mg PO). They were then randomized into a blinded, placebo-controlled, double cross-over study. Group A received placebo for 8 weeks, followed by repeat MRI with hypercapnia challenge, followed by 8 weeks of sildenafil, 25 mg twice daily orally. Group B received the sildenafil first, followed by repeat MRI, and then 8 weeks of placebo. We also had a group of 20 healthy control participants and a group of 20 recovered TBI participants without symptoms, all of whom under-went the MRI with hypercapnia BOLD at baseline, with and without a single dose of sildenafil (50 mg PO).

We were particularly interested in the relationship between these vascular imaging biomarkers and the patients' symptoms. Our primary objective was to deter-mine if single-dose treatment with sildenafil (50 mg orally) would be effective in increasing regional and global BOLD response to hypercapnia in symptomatic patients in the chronic stage after TBI. Sildenafil safety and tolerability at these doses in this population were secondary objectives.

Participant Demographics

Table 12.1 shows the demographics of the participants in the study. We studied a total of 35 TBI subjects, combining together the symptomatic and recovered TBI subjects for the purpose of this analysis. The aver-age age was about 40, and they were mostly males. These were civilian TBIs from car accidents and falls. We had a well-educated group of people. The TBI folks

TABLE 12.1
Participant Demographics

	TBI (n=35)	HC (n=20)	P
Age (years), mean±STD	39.0±9.0	37.5±8.9	ns
Gender, % male	77	80	ns
Education (years), median (IQR)	15 (13–18)	17 (14–19)	.064
NBSI, median (IQR)	11 (6–19)	3 (1–6)	<.001

HC, healthy control participants; *IQR*, interquartile range; *NBSI*, neurobehavioral symptom inventory; *STD*, standard deviation; *TBI*, participants with traumatic brain injury.

were symptomatic but not hugely symptomatic: their neurobehavioral symptom inventory score was in the medium range, about 11 on average. They had their TBI about 3 years prior to the study, with the majority (55%) being due to car accidents. Thirty-seven percent had a loss of conciseness longer than 30 min, so most had a complicated mild to moderate TBI, and most were admitted to the hospital overnight. The median time in the intensive care unit was 3 days, and a little more than one-third received inpatient rehabilitation.

Assessment of Vessel Reactivity With CO_2

This is how we did the study: the patient is placed in the MRI magnet and connected to a bag that is filled with 5% carbon dioxide, which is a potent vasodila-tor. Every minute, the gas that the patient breathes is switched from room air to 5% carbon dioxide and that is enough to elevate the end tidal CO_2 approximately 10 mm Hg, from about 40 to about 50 mm Hg. This is a technique that has been used for decades to assess vascular reactivity, and in the magnet we can follow the end tidal CO_2 and also the blood oxygenation level-dependent (BOLD) MRI signal. The BOLD signal is a good way to assess the ability of the vessel to deliver more blood flow, and you can then map the blood flow in a pixel-by-pixel manner throughout the whole brain.

Assessment of Cerebral Blood Flow Using Arterial Spin Labeling and Cerebrovascular Reactivity Using Hypercapnia BOLD MRI

Fig. 12.8 shows the basic finding of this study. In healthy individuals, the cerebral blood flows assessed either through arterial spin labeling (ASL) or through cerebrovascular reactivity (CVR) is uniform. The blood flow and CVR are not uniform, however, after a TBI. You can see in Fig. 12.8 two different patients who are representative of our TBI sample. The patient "b" in the

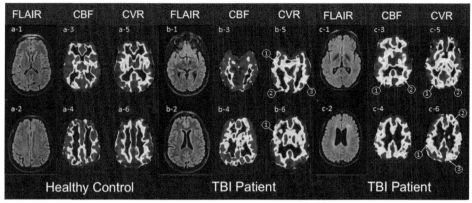

FIG. 12.8 Assessment of cerebral blood flow (CBF) with arterial spin labeling and cerebrovascular reactivity (CVR) with hypercapnia blood oxygenation level-dependent MRI. *FLAIR*, fluid-attenuated inversion recovery; *TBI*, traumatic brain injury. (Figure courtesy of Dr. Diaz-Arrastia.)

middle panels had a normal T2 fluid-attenuated inversion recovery (FLAIR) MRI showing no visible abnormalities, yet on the cerebral blood flow (CBF) map we do see a "moth eaten" appearance with "holes" of decreased CBF scattered in many parts of the brain, and when we measure CVR we notice that there are even more abnormalities—many more "holes" in the CVR map, indicating poor cerebrovascular reactivity in those regions. Patient "c" in the rightmost panels has subtle areas of damage, including T2 FLAIR abnormalities and encephalomalacia, and, as expected, there are corresponding abnormalities in the CBF and CVR, but we also see many more "holes" in these maps that are not detectable on standard clinical MRI scans.

Fig. 12.9 shows another way to look at CVR and CBF using statistical voxel-based nonparametric mapping techniques. The images show voxels that are at least two standard deviations different from the pool of healthy controls, and we can identify these "holes" in both the CBF and CVR maps. When we look at the overall statistics of every voxel in the brain, although there are differences between the TBI patients and controls for CBF ($P = .04$, Cohen's $d = 0.68$), the difference is much more pronounced for CVR ($P < .001$, Cohen's $d = 0.90$). Interestingly, the relationship between resting CBF and CVR is actually quite weak.

Single-Dose Sildenafil in Patients With Chronic TBI and Healthy Controls

Not only did CVR distinguish between patients with chronic TBI and controls much better that CBF, but we also found that CVR was even more different between patients and controls when we took the patients out of the MRI and gave them a single 50-mg dose of sildenafil, waited an hour, and put them back in the MRI to look for potentiation of the CVR by sildenafil. In control individuals basically nothing happened—in fact, there was slight decrease, which is surprising at first but it has been known for decades that there is some desensitization of vasculature to the hypercapnia stimulus, which is probably what we are seeing. On the other hand, when we gave sildenafil to the TBI patients, almost every case showed an increase in the CVR and the results were highly statically significant (Fig. 12.10).

Looking in at the maps in Fig. 12.11 is somewhat instructive. The increase in cerebrovascular reactivity is not global—it doesn't occur everywhere in the brain—it is specific to some of those "holes." Fig. 12.11 shows one patient who had very visible T2 FLAIR abnormalities in the right temporal lobe as well as some encephalomalacia. As expected, there are "holes" in the CBF and CVR maps associated with the FLAIR abnormalities and the encephalomalacia. There are also many "holes" in the CBF and CVR that are not associated with these anatomical abnormalities. When we give these patients sildenafil, not much happens in the area that has encephalomalacia. On the other hand, immediately adjacent to that and many other areas as well there is potentiation of the CVR as a consequence of sildenafil.

We also found that the CVR is weakly correlated with some aspects of cognitive function. We were hoping for more, but it's a small study and we can't complain about what the data show. Anecdotally, we did notice that, although this was a placebo-controlled double-blind trial (so that neither the patient nor us knew what drug they were taking during a particular 8-week period), we asked them when they came in after 8 weeks, "Are you better?" and, if

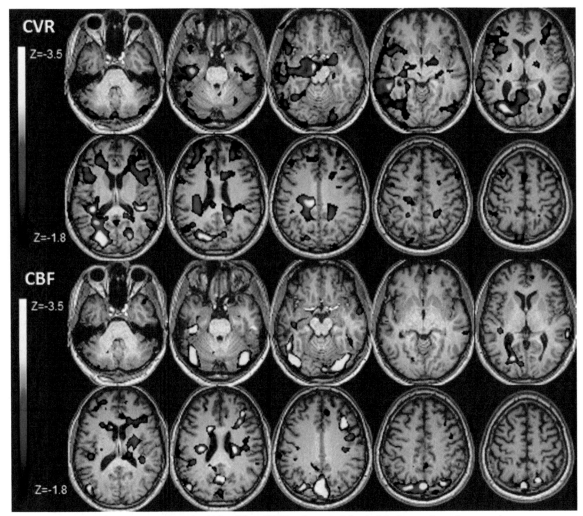

FIG. 12.9 Assessment of cerebral blood flow (CBF) using arterial spin labeling and cerebrovascular reactivity (CVR) using hypercapnia blood oxygenation level-dependent MRI analyzed with statistical voxel-based nonparametric mapping techniques. The images show voxels that are at least two standard deviations different from the pool of healthy controls. (Figure courtesy of Dr. Diaz-Arrastia.)

you're better, "Are you a little better, a lot better, or much improved?" and a subset of the patients—about nine—told us that they were at least somewhat better and about seven said they were better during a sildenafil phase. This finding is not significant, so I don't want to make a big deal about it, but I can say at the dose we tried these folks tolerated sildenafil very well. We were worried about headache, as it is one of the main side effects of sildenafil, and many of these patients had headache at baseline, and we were worried that the sildenafil would make their headache worse, but it was not case.

FUNCTIONAL NEAR-INFRARED SPECTROSCOPY

We are developing another technique that measures CVR, and we are optimistic about it. Our MRI techniques are very good at measuring CVR and CBF, but they are expensive, cumbersome, and not well suited for bedside or clinic-based testing, so we studied functional near-infrared spectroscopy (fNIRS), and the results are promising (Fig. 12.12). There is a good correlation between using the BOLD fMRI and fNIRS to measure CVR, both in individual subjects and across a group (Fig. 12.13).

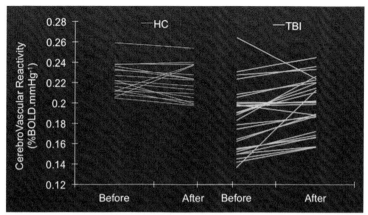

FIG. 12.10 Single-dose sildenafil potentiates cerebrovascular reactivity in patients with chronic traumatic brain injury (TBI) but not in healthy controls (HC). *BOLD*, blood oxygenation level-dependent MRI. (Figure courtesy of Dr. Diaz-Arrastia.)

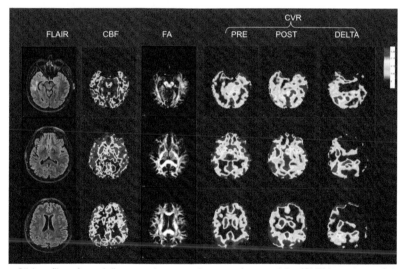

FIG. 12.11 Sildenafil preferentially potentiates cerebrovascular reactivity (CVR) in regions of damaged endothelium. The images show standard T2 fluid-attenuated inversion recovery MRI, as well as assessment of cerebral blood flow (CBF) using arterial spin labeling and CVR using hypercapnia blood oxygenation level-dependent MRI analyzed with statistical voxel-based nonparametric mapping techniques. (Figure courtesy of Dr. Diaz-Arrastia.)

CONCLUSIONS

So in conclusion, I hope I made a case that we are going to need biomarkers in order to rationally design the next generation of clinical trials in TBI, and the first generation of trials in CTE. We think that for TBI, CVR shows promise as pharmacodynamic biomarker of traumatic microvascular injury, at least in the population that we studied. Whether it is also a predictive biomarker will require further study. Sildenafil is well

tolerated at 25 mg BID (twice a day) in patients with chronic TBI, and it improves the regional CVR deficits in these patients.

There are still many remaining questions. What is the role of sildenafil in the acute and subacute stage after TBI? Is there a benefit of sildenafil in mild TBI? Is there a role for sildenafil in older patients with TBI? In our study, the age cut off was 55 because we didn't want to be confounded by the well-known effect of age on

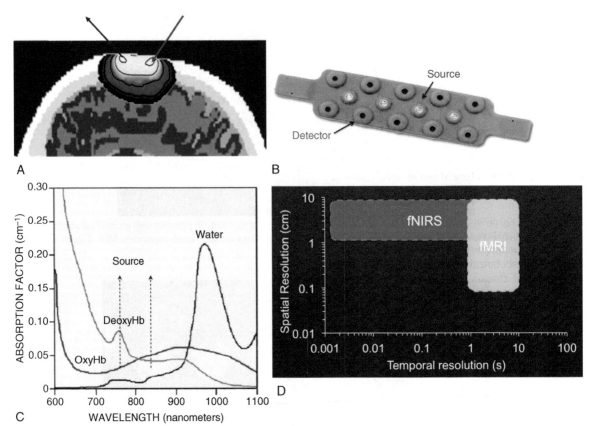

A

B

C

D

FIG. 12.12 Functional near-infrared spectroscopy (fNIRS). **(A)** The source of the near-infrared light is directed from the scalp to the surface of the cortex, and then the reflected light is detected by the sensor. **(B)** An example of the fNIRS equipment used. It is placed on the forehead. **(C)** fNIRS uses light waves that can detect oxygenated and deoxygenated hemoglobin. **(D)** Compared with functional MRI (fMRI), fNIRS has worse spatial resolution but better temporal resolution, lower cost, and greater portability. (Figure courtesy of Franck Amyot, CNRM/NICHD.)

CVR. Is CVR a useful predictive biomarker? Can fNIRS replace or complement BOLD fMRI as a tool measuring CVR? Are there blood biomarkers of microvascular injury? What is the relationship between CBF, CVR, and blood-brain barrier integrity? And finally, we want to investigate the relationship between traumatic microvascular injury and traumatic axonal injury. These are often talked about interchangeably, but I would suspect they are not exactly the same.

All of this work was done in Bethesda, at the NIH Clinical Center, and we are getting it set up at the University of Pennsylvania. I want to thank all of my colleagues and collaborators. Thank you very much for your attention.

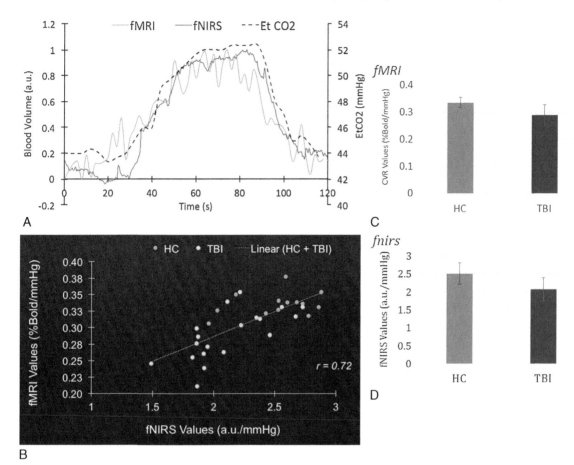

FIG. 12.13 Functional near-infrared spectroscopy (fNIRS) versus functional MRI (fMRI). **(A)** For the same subject, under the same CO_2 challenge, both fNIRS and the blood oxygenation level-dependent (BOLD) signal with fMRI give a similar hemodynamic response function. The hemodynamic response functions for fNIRS and fMRI follow the same trend as the end-tidal carbon dioxide (EtCO2). **(B)** Correlation of BOLD fMRI with fNIRS for cerebrovascular reactivity across a group of healthy controls (HC) and subjects with traumatic brain injury (TBI). **(C)** Group differences detected using fMRI. Effect size (Cohen's d) = 2.3; $P < .0001$. **(D)** Group differences detected using fNIRS. Effect size (Cohen's d) = 1.3; $P < .0001$. TBI, traumatic brain injury. (Figure courtesy of Franck Amyot, CNRM/NICHD.)

REFERENCES

1. Almasy L, Blangero J. Endophenotypes as quantitative risk factors for psychiatric disease: rationale and study design. *American Journal of Medical Genetics.* January 8, 2001;105(1):42–44.
2. Robb MA, McInnes PM, Califf RM. Biomarkers and surrogate endpoints: developing common terminology and definitions. *JAMA.* March 15, 2016;315(11):1107–1108. http://dx.doi.org/10.1001/jama.2016.2240.
3. Zlokovic BV. Neurovascular pathways to neurodegeneration in Alzheimer's disease and other disorders. *Nature Reviews. Neuroscience.* November 3, 2011;12(12):723–738. http://dx.doi.org/10.1038/nrn3114.
4. Weber B, Keller AL, Reichold J, Logothetis NK. The microvascular system of the striate and extrastriate visual cortex of the macaque. *Cerebral Cortex.* October 2008;18(10): 2318–2330. http://dx.doi.org/10.1093/cercor/bhm259.
5. Graham DI, Lantos PL, eds. *Greenfield's Neuropathology.* 7th ed. London: Arnold; 2002.
6. Maxwell WL, Irvine A, Adams JH, Graham DI, Gennarelli TA. Response of cerebral microvasculature to brain injury. *The Journal of Pathology.* August 1988;155(4):327–335.
7. Rodriguez-Baeza A, Reina-De La Torre F, Ortega-Sanchez M, Sahuquillo-Barris J. Perivascular structures in corrosion casts of the human central nervous system: a confocal laser and scanning electron microscope study. *The Anatomical Record.* October 1998;252(2):176–184.

8. Rodríguez-Baeza A, Reina-de la Torre F, Poca A, Martí M, Garnacho A. Morphological features in human cortical brain microvessels after head injury: a three-dimensional and immunocytochemical study. *The Anatomical Record. Part A, Discoveries in Molecular, Cellular, and Evolutionary Biology*. July 2003;273(1):583–593.

9. Ding G, Jiang Q, Li L, et al. Magnetic resonance imaging investigation of axonal remodeling and angiogenesis after embolic stroke in sildenafil-treated rats. *Journal of Cerebral Blood Flow and Metabolism*. August 2008;28(8):1440–1448. http://dx.doi.org/10.1038/jcbfm.2008.33.

10. Weissberg I, Veksler R, Kamintsky L, et al. Imaging blood–brain barrier dysfunction in football players. *JAMA Neurology*. November 2014;71(11):1453–1455. http://dx.doi.org/10.1001/jamaneurol.2014.2682.

CHAPTER 13

Athlete Panel Discussion

CHRISTOPHER J. NOWINSKI

Note: Although introduced by name at the conference, in this chapter one athlete chose to remain anonymous. Certain details have been changed or omitted to protect his privacy.

Mr. Christopher Nowinski: Thank you Dr. Budson, and thank you to everyone for being here and learning from this great group of doctors. I am Chris Nowinski, and I am here with three esteemed panelists. I will introduce them after I give some brief information about our foundation.

For those of you who don't know me, I got into this work back in 2003 when I got hit in the head too much. We thought since we will have a chronic traumatic encephalopathy (CTE) athlete patient panel we would have a CTE moderator. I played football for Harvard and wrestled for World Wrestling Entertainment (WWE). I got concussed out of WWE in 2003, and I was diagnosed with postconcussion syndrome by Dr. Robert Cantu (Chapter 1). Dr. Cantu inspired me to try to change the way we deal with concussions because, from my own ignorance, it was playing through every concussion I ever had. That probably led to my postconcussion syndrome.

THE CONCUSSION LEGACY FOUNDATION

The way we look at ourselves now, in part we are the recruiters for the brain bank. We are recruiting for Dr. Ann McKee, Dr. Thor Stein, and their team, so they can do their great research. Then we try to translate those findings into how we can protect the athletes. A lot of that is policy and advocacy work. For example, we worked hard to successfully get heading out of soccer before age 11 through our Safer Soccer Initiative. We are working on getting a lot of the hitting out of football practice. We have a new education program called Team Up & Speak Up, in which we are teaching athletes to look after their teammates on the field. We have other education programs as well. Especially around the Boston area we do a lot of lectures for kids. The 30-min Team Up Against Concussion program goes to the schools to educate children, and speakers do trainings for coaches and for all sorts of folks through our Advanced Concussion Training program. So please use us. Feel free to reach out to me at ConcussionFoundation.org. We bring training and consulting services to help everything from schools to cities. We are currently working in the city of Somerville, Massachusetts, and we are going to do some radical things over there. Anyways, it's an honor to work with these guys, and to try and accelerate that process from knowledge to practice.

INTRODUCTION OF THE PANEL

So with that I will transition to these three stars who were willing to join me for this panel. I will start by saying that we are calling this the "CTE patient panel" in the conference. But we never actually had a discussion around how you know who has CTE since there is no definitive clinical diagnosis. So I decided to invite three guys who, like me, have probably hit their head too much and are knowledgeable about this topic and are willing talk about their own experiences. None of us know exactly what's going on in our heads, but we have our suspicions, and so we are going to share with you what we know. I will prompt some questions, but it's really about what you want to learn from them. So if you start writing down your own questions we will have time to answer them.

I will start to my near side. Most of you will recognize Tim Fox who, after graduating from The Ohio State, was a first round draft pick with the Patriots and played in the National Football League for 11 seasons as a safety. He recently went public with his concerns about CTE.

To his right is the great Kevin McBride. He was a 1992 Olympic Boxer for Ireland with a career record of 35 wins, 10 losses, and 1 tie. Most of you, like me, remember him for knocking out Mike Tyson in 2005. I ran into him at Boston Medical Center (BMC) (his wife works there), and I got him to pledge me his brain in the coffee line of Starbucks. Since then we have been close friends.

And to his right is another former NFL player who retired 10 years ago. In his 8 years in the NFL he played for multiple teams. On special teams, he was a wedge buster, which is a position known for incredible collisions.

I appreciate you guys being here. I will start with you, Tim. You recently went public with some of your concerns, so tell these folks what you have been feeling and what you think it means?

Mr. Tim Fox: Well, first off, people talk about how it's great you're letting people know about your concerns, but frankly, I don't see this as a stigma associated with myself. Over the last 10 years or so I noticed a significant decline in my recognition capabilities—remembering names, remembering where I put things, remembering where I am going. It gets to the point where it's embarrassing when you're out in public and you meet people you know you know, and you can't think for the life of you of what their names are. But more concerning is that I can't remember where I met them. So, it's something I feel that is very important and we need to bring attention to it.

I think we need to make changes in youth sports to make sure people understand the jeopardy they are in and take steps to avoid those problems. In my career, I played 12 years in the NFL, so when you add it all together with college, high school, and Pop Warner, it's 20-something years of getting hit in the head.

You always wonder if it is normal aging, but it's frustrating when you talk to people and you start to share your story and they say, "I am the same way, I can't remember where I put my keys," and I get that, but when you get to the point that you can no longer do your daily functions, I would argue that it is different. I just recently retired, a month ago, from a financial company in which I was in a very stressful position. It just got to the point where I was scared to death that I was going to forget to call someone back or put an order in. It weighs you down. So I am out of that business, and I am doing everything I can to try to bring more awareness to this disease.

Mr. Nowinski: Thank you Tim. Kevin, how is your head feeling? We haven't even talked about it yet.

Mr. Kevin McBride: Hello everybody! My name is Kevin and Chris is my translator because I am Irish. Listen, it is a pleasure to be around these guys and help people find the problems caused by brain trauma and all that stuff. I've been boxing since I was 9 years old and probably before that. I went professional and started winning fights. I like boxing because of the buzz you get when you knock someone out, but when you get knocked out yourself you get a different buzz. I did get knocked out a few times.

My last fight I woke up in the hospital and I said "Jesus," because I was in the hospital and I didn't remember the night of the fight or the week before and few days after. Then for maybe a few months after the fight when I would jump out of bed to see my kids—I have two beautiful kids—I had to hold the wall because my equilibrium was messed up. So I had to walk along the wall to pull myself together.

Like Tim was saying, I also forget where my keys are. I do tree work now, and a few days ago I forget where I was. If I really think I can go back in time but I still couldn't remember how I got here, if my boss drove me here or this is where I was; it's hard to remember. My daughter is now 12 but when she was 3 or 4 she used to make fun of me by saying, "da da da daddy," and she was mocking me and my stutter and we laughed. It's funny, but it's probably because of boxing.

Mr. Nowinski: I appreciate all of you telling us those things, and I know all the doctors at the conference appreciate it as well. I didn't push any of you guys to reveal more than what you are comfortable with, but I can tell that you will keep revealing a lot and I appreciate it and your willingness to talk about this issue. So we talked a lot about memory as a symptom, and that's always the first thing to think about. But we know now from the scientific work that there are other symptoms related to CTE as well. Some of you talked about depression, and there is a lot of research around impulse control issues as well. Are these symptoms something any of you are seeing in your own life or among your peers?

Mr. Fox: There is no question but that you can look at a series of symptoms for CTE and you can just go down and check off the boxes. In my case, when I look at all the symptoms, I check "yes, yes, yes, yes," and then at some point you think am I being a hypochondriac and I am assuming the worst. Let me tell you about something that may get a little bit off the topic here. One of the things I went in to have checked because of my history of head trauma is my pituitary gland, which lies behind your forehead and is very susceptible to head injury. So the endocrinologist puts you through a series of tests where they inject you with something and there are 3 h with sitting in a chair and they draw blood every 15 min to see if your pituitary gland is secreting what it's supposed to secrete. It turns out that mine is secreting absolutely no human growth hormone. There are three things that may cause an adult to have a pituitary gland problem. You either have a pituitary tumor, a brain tumor, or head trauma. So you go through another series of tests with brain scans to make sure you don't have a tumor and you're left with the obvious choice, which is head trauma. And the problem with that is that the lack of human growth hormone in you produces symptoms that are similar to symptoms of CTE, including loss of memory, your tolerance for people around you, and so it's frustrating.

Some of these guys that Dr. McKee (Chapter 2) and Dr. Stern (Chapter 3) talked about were young guys—well, younger than me. At 55-years-old, after playing for 12 years, I am thinking, "I got through the game of football pretty good." I feel all right. Then I hear about all these horror stories that in that next 5 to 10 years there may be a marked decrease in my cognitive ability. I also had a hip replaced, knee replaced, and a shoulder replaced. And now I am not sure I got through the game all that well. For me, I was willing to buy in for the physical injuries. I knew that I could injure my knee or hurt my hip and shoulders. But those things can be fixed, and they have been fixed. All is working well, and I am doing the things I want to do. But we have to figure out how to fix the head, because I didn't buy into that.

Mr. McBride: The brain is precious and life is precious, and you have to take it day by day. When I leave here I will forget where I park my car. It's crazy, but I am just hoping people will understand the traumatic effects of trauma or whatever you call that word.

NFL Player: I also want to say that as a man from a group of men who are not into admitting any weaknesses that being in an atmosphere of what Chris has created is incredible. That atmosphere hasn't previously existed.

Mr. Nowinski: Tim, what are the concerns among your community and the people you played with?

Mr. Fox: I have several friends with concerns, some worse than me and some not as bad as me. You feel like it's a ticking time bomb, and you don't know how long the fuse is. I think the work Chris and the Boston University folks have done has brought attention to these concerns. That needed to be done, and now there are changes in the game. When I played, we tried to knock people out. For us, that was the easiest way to get the guy out of the game, because, in our minds, he was unconscious, but he would come back out and play the next week. Nobody wanted to physically hurt someone such that they would have to have surgery, and we thought knocking someone out was the goal. We would watch the films and, man, when you saw the big hits the room would go, "oh man!" It was a badge of honor that you could do that.

Now you see changes in the NFL, and it needs to trickle down to high school, Pop Warner, and college: you can't leave the decision to go back into the game up to the player, because in the NFL that is how people make their living and that's the only thing they are good at for the rest of their life. The difference between good players and great players is opportunity. So if you're playing and you go down and you leave the game with a concussion, and the guy behind you goes in and makes an interception and has a good game, all of a sudden those roles reversed, and he is playing and you're on the bench and you can't feed your family. So it's important that the NFL takes that decision away from the players. They have a concussion protocol now and we didn't have that. Our protocol was: they would take you to the sidelines, give you smelling salts, and ask you your phone number, and put you back in the game. And your buddy would usually give you your phone number, and the doctor would say, "close enough," and back in you would go.

Mr. Nowinski: Kevin, do boxers talk about that?

Mr. McBride: Boxing is a fun sport, just like people play football for the good buzz. Sometimes I think about my son and boxing. I haven't taught him yet.

Mr. Nowinski: Do you think you will teach him at a certain age?

Mr. McBride: I think it's his own decision, but I try to not encourage it. It's tough because people have died doing this sport and people die in football too. Listen, I've had opportunities but I know after you get knocked out you can't box for a month or so. But behind closed doors there is all that sparring. You don't know that people are probably getting CTE. Someone might not know. For me, when you get older, now I have to write things down so I know won't forget them.

Mr. Nowinski: How about you, NFL Player, are your buddies talking about this?

NFL Player: I think the other important aspects are the changes made to the game. These are changes that needed to be made for football to survive and everyone needs to follow suit, which is reducing the impact to the lowest impact. One thing Chris talks about is acknowledging that issue, so it is important to take away the impacts in practice. I don't need to practice hitting my head to get good at it—it's ridiculous. And 85% of impacts come from practice, which is ridiculous. This idea of taking a hit or taking a punch is ludicrous. There are safe ways to practice, and right there you're taking a huge chunk of impact exposure off table. The crucial problem is not about just the NFL, it is about the sport all the way down to the college, high school, and Pop Warner levels; they all need to implement the right rules. Let's be honest, football is a violent sport.

Mr. Nowinski: How was your football game last night?

NFL Player: I coach my son's middle school football team. He is 13 years old. We played a team. Long story short, we showed up at an away game, our sixth and seventh graders were supposed to play sixth and seventh graders from another school. So we showed up, and I could tell right when I got off the bus that there was no way the players on their team were in sixth and seventh grade. They looked huge. I went over to the coach and asked how old they were, and whether they were in sixth and seventh grade, and he said, "no, we are all eighth graders." I was like yeah, that doesn't feel right to me, and I talked to the coach and said we probably won't play this game.

But it was a 45-min bus ride and so we negotiated that maybe we will see how it goes with our guys on the seventh grade team and his second and third string group, and we agreed to that. The game starts and their kids don't look like seventh graders moving the ball. So they are up two touchdowns we have a meeting to stop the game and I said we should call this and leave because this doesn't feel safe for my son or the team and the parents are trusting me with their kids. And I asked them one more time, saying, "hey, I gave you the opportunity," and "can we please try this again?" And he said, "yes." So this made a difference and we got to fourth down and we said, "alright, perfect, he will punt the ball."

But just as I said, "this feels safer," he shuffles in his first string team, goes for it, and one of our guys gets hurt on the play. I flipped out. I walked onto the field and I said a few choice words. I don't like losing my temper, but I said a few choice words and pulled our whole team and called the bus driver and we walked right out of there with some ridicule from the fans telling us we were bad sports without understanding the story that it was about the safety of the kids. It's a long story that probably wouldn't have happened in a varsity sport—then you would have to tough it out and get through it—but there was no way we were going to do it with sixth and seventh graders. I got an email before I got here today from the athletic director, which said that all the parents said, "thank you," to the coaching staff and me for looking after their kids.

Mr. Nowinski: I could ask the panel more questions, but it's more about what you in the conference want to learn, so I want to go to the audience and I will start with a question from Dr. McKee.

Dr. Ann McKee: I am curious if your symptoms decrease if you exercise, and if you feel better if your symptoms are improved.

NFL Player: Yeah, you are probably asking that for a reason. There is no doubt that making exercise a priority makes every single person in this room feel better. I think there is marked improvement with

exercise in my experience as well. The problem is that we have the usual issue of being moms and parents and not always having enough time. I think your point is a good one: the focus on energy, diet, and fitness should be a high priority, and even more so in a situation like this.

Dr. McKee: Do you notice that headaches are less or sleep is better or anything like that?

Mr. Nowinski: For me, exercise makes me feel better. More energy, a higher level of endurance over time. Not big highs and big lows, not big crashes. I'll note that sometimes when you are an ex-athlete it can be hard to exercise due to previous injuries.

NFL Player: Yeah, I have to get two knee replacements and so currently I have to get my exercise from walking. I was a spaz when I played, and there is no outlet quite like that now. I can cycle now and I guess that's close. But you're limited in your choice of exercise. I walk around in pain every day and that wears on me over time.

Mr. Fox: I think there is no question that exercise and staying active not only helps you physically but also mentally. It gives you something to look forward to and gives you a competitive spirit, but you can't exercise at the level you want to because of your knees, etc. I would love to play tennis but I can't. It scares me with all of the artificial stuff in my body. You try to stay active. It tends to be a lot of walking and playing with the kids and grandkids.

Mr. Nowinski: Kevin, you still punching people?

Mr. McBride: No, thank God. I love boxing because I grew up with it and I love it and I loved it when I was in shape. The buzz when you were in the ring, the power, it's all great. When I was boxing, a guy like me—you change because you got a big head—you want to rip their head off and then when you do you hope they are ok. When I hit Mike Tyson in the sixth round he hit me back so hard I thought there were leprechauns playing in my head. Everyone knows when you're in shape and you feel good and you feel on top of the world, but as far as getting punches to the head it's not good, that's why we are here. I had a lot of impacts to my head from tough guys. I got hit so hard I thought I was in Ireland and I was really in America. I thank God I am alive. My wife is a nurse, and there is no way she would put gloves on our kids. My girl punches well though; she would knock you out!

Dr. Jesse Mez: So, regarding contact sports, what do you recommend to teams or those who are boxing who are at the cusp of entering sports at the high school level? What are your recommendations? Do it? Or don't do it? Or do it safer?

Mr. McBride: This is a man's—and a woman's—world and you want to be the best at whatever you do and you want to dream. You would love to see them go into the sport they love. People want to see the sport use head guards for boxing. They are not really that good because when you get hit it still shakes the brain, although maybe it's better. You would push them on to do the best in whatever they do and hopefully they'll get more protective equipment and if you get a concussion you get the right amount of time off and you don't get back into the ring right away. But I don't think you will ever be 100% safe, but that's the sport we live in and I love it. We just need more resources so they don't get hurt as much.

Mr. Fox: I think football is a great game. I played for a college coach by the name of Woody Hayes; he used to say you would learn more on the football field than you would in any classroom about life. And I agree. However, there is risk associated with that. I have a son who is now 29 and he wanted to play Pop Warner at age 11 and I went to the league and told them he wanted to play and they said, "that's great." I said, "I have had some experience with football if you need help with coaching," and they said, "thanks, we're all set," and they took him even though he was entering this group when he was age 11, and others had been playing since they were 8 years old. He would get a little time to play but then we moved for more opportunities to Westwood. He played at Boston College on a full scholarship and broke his ankle twice and collarbone once and he only played 1 year. After graduating, he wanted to try out in the NFL and asked me to help. And I said, "no way that I am pulling that string for you. If you couldn't stay healthy playing at the collegiate level you can't stay healthy for the NFL." For people who want their kids to play in Pop Warner I say, "yes," but you need to go there and watch them and see if you agree with what they are doing, and if you don't agree, then you need to speak up.

NFL Player: I would never let my son play if they wouldn't let me coach. Tim, I think your message is right. I have seen really terrible coaching and my playing a role is the reason why my son is playing now. I would not trust others to coach him. To your question about sports, Dr. Mez, I thought long and hard about this. Sports are woven into America. Sports are competitive, and we have contact sports not just in America but in other countries as well. On the other hand, I wrote a case study on this issue, how contact sports are woven into our country uniquely. There is an obsession with sports, and it goes hand in hand with the idea of being a student and an athlete. There are so many lessons on

both sides, and having a well-rounded upbringing is important. Now playing safely is everyone's goal, and every single league needs to be focused on that. Obviously, Chris is driving toward that. There is risk with any contact sport, and the solution is not yanking competitive and contact sports, it's making them safer and creating an environment that you feel safe enough to admit when you have symptoms. That's changing, but it needs to change even more.

I've got to run now to another appointment, but I want to thank you for inviting me, and for all the important work that you all are doing.

Dr. Andrew Budson: I want to thank all of you for talking to us. A lot of us here in the room are very interested in trying to figure out what are the symptoms and what happens after you have had so many head hits. And we talked about it generally, but I would love for each of you to give one example, whether it's something you forgot, you couldn't pay attention to, or if you were irritable and you think it's probably from all the hits you had.

Mr. Fox: I see a change in my personality and my tolerance toward things, including a change in my emotions and my patience. If my wife were here, she would give 1700 examples of that. Emotionally, I used to be very stoic. I was sharing with Dr. Stern that my wife and I lost three parents last year. I lost my dad 20 years ago, and at that time I was able to speak at his funeral and go through the scenario and it was what it was. Flashing forward to last year, I couldn't even speak at the recent funerals. I was so overcome by emotion that I couldn't do it. I don't know exactly what has changed, but there was a big difference.

Mr. McBride: My wife would tell you a millions things. She would say you think you did this and that when you didn't, and especially da da da—my stutter. I am more aware now that the stutter must be from boxing because everyone in my family talks fine. Every day is a challenge because you do forget things. I notice more now that I am 43 years old. Comparing a couple years ago to now I forget things more. I don't know if that's from boxing or something else, and I only remember 2 years of being in this country. I just don't remember. I know, for instance, everybody forgets where they put their keys, and a good decision was to put my keys on the key rack. But then I still don't know where the keys are. My wife gets mad because I look for the keys, and she says they're on the rack. There is also a factor with remembering names and all that stuff. I could know your face but I can't remember your name.

I met Muhammad Ali after I beat Mike Tyson because he wanted to say goodbye and I gave him a hug and a hand shake and he said, "you're the latest and I am the greatest." It was great just to meet him. I got pictures. Everyone here, if you want to talk to my wife, there is a documentary and a guy followed me around after I beat Mike Tyson and I was bashed up with black and blues and it shows the traumatic effects of boxing. Thank God doctors are in the room to discover things.

For example, I needed to do a written test and I needed to study and I thought there was no way that I could remember. And I kept reading and I kept practicing the test and I read for 5 or 6 h the night before. I passed the general knowledge test and they give me the paper. I passed and I was so excited that I am not as stupid as I sometimes think. I think maybe there are some brain cells—not too many—and I am still learning and life is brilliant as far as your brain goes. Sometimes I have no clue what I do or say but I wish you all the best of luck!

Audience Question: I am curious. So, if Dr. Stern (or anyone else) had a test that could give you maybe 90% confidence that you do or don't have CTE—but there's still no treatment for it—would you take the test now or wait until there is a treatment?

Mr. Fox: I would definitely want to know. The problem with the cognitive test they can give you now is that if you don't have a baseline then they don't know where you fall on the cognitive spectrum. Of course, everyone thinks they're smart—and I was probably stupid—but going through The Ohio State I graduated. I mean, to be honest, I read the books but I didn't study. I read them and I passed the test. If I try to do that today my performance would be nonexistent. Now I have to read things over and over again and I probably would still forget. I would want the test to know (A) I am not crazy and (B) I am not imagining things. I want to solve the problem.

Mr. McBride: At the end of passing the test if someone asked me the material I wouldn't have a clue. If it would help football players and boxers, I wouldn't mind going for the test to help my kids or future generations—as long as you give me a few perks. (laughs) Honest to God, it's all new to me. It would be great if you can go to the doctor's office and be sick mentally and he or she gives you a tablet and says, "here, take this and you will be fine," and you take the tablets and a week later you're back on the top of the world because you think the pill makes you better. And I know you people are trying to figure it out and it's all science. You have to come up with a cure to help me remember. I want to enjoy life.

Audience Question: My question is for Chris. Do you reach out to current NFL players? Are they hesitant or are they willing to get involved in donating their brains?

Mr. Nowinski: I've talked to five active NFL players and, in general, they are purposely avoiding this issue. They don't want to be labeled a "concussion guy" and lose money in their next contract negotiation.

Mr. McBride: I am sure if you are making money you don't want to say you have a concussion because you like the money.

Mr. Nowinski: I would note that it is rare that people are talking as openly as they are doing today on this panel. This doesn't happen very often, but today we have some nice guys who were willing to do it.

Dr. Lee Goldstein: Thank you all. We are grateful for the opportunity to hear the story from the inside. I am astonished—I shouldn't be—that this is the response of the active players in the NFL. I am wondering if that sort of mentality is also true at the collegiate or amateur elite level, or is it more or less unique to professional athletes.

Mr. Fox: You're in the game because you want to play the game, and if you say you have an issue you won't play. And so many kids at the collegiate level want to play in the NFL and make millions and if you start saying you have head injuries, it goes in the record and on draft day you go down the list. So from a financial standpoint it is not in your best interest. From health standpoint it is, but at that age you can't force them to worry about their health.

Mr. Nowinski: I think this issue is not part of their education. They get told about concussions, but CTE education is not required. If they read a recent issue of a National Collegiate Athletic Association (NCAA) produced magazine, they'll hear NCAA doctors saying this CTE stuff is overblown. The one note that is interesting is Christine Baugh surveyed NCAA football players, and 10% said they are concerned about CTE. That's all we know.

Audience Question: How did the negotiations happen that NFL practice time was reduced? Where did that pressure come from?

Mr. Nowinski: We showed them the data. We got 5 min to talk at the first NFLPA Mackey-White Health & Safety Committee meeting to give one big idea that would help. We were the only ones who pointed out that we can take out 67% of the hits that lead to concussions if you shorten practice, and the players said, "yeah that's stupid, we hate that, we will back that." The sad fact was that the NFL players had to negotiate for their own health and had to give up money for less hitting in practice. That's sick.

Audience Question: How about the pushback of coaches are saying that the games are worse because they don't practice enough?

Mr. Nowinski: My personal opinion is that it's a new convenient excuse to blame for poor performance.

Audience Question: So I want to jump back to Mr. Fox's comment that if you went through a battery of neurocognitive testing it wouldn't be helpful because you don't know the baseline and so you wouldn't know if the results changed. So do you think baseline neurocognitive testing should be implemented for kids and high school athletes in order to track their cognitive functioning so if they continue playing you can retest them and compare it to their baseline? Would that be helpful?

Mr. Fox: The NFL test is given to rookies, and I think that is important so you know where you are. However, there is a broad spectrum of normal, and if you start at the top and go to the bottom of the normal spectrum, that may be more significant than if you were at the bottom and dropped just a little out of range. As long as you test within those guidelines the way the NFL does it, it's hard to say what's wrong with you.

Audience Question: We heard a lot about football in the United States, but can you say something in terms of advocacy around the world?

Mr. Nowinski: The rest of the world is behind us. English-speaking countries are starting to have their opinions heard, but beyond that it gets thin. For example, there are no discussions regarding whether headers are appropriate for kids from the Fédération Internationale de Football Association (FIFA). We don't have the rest of the world mobilized. Some people have begun looking for CTE postmortem in Scotland, Brazil, and Australia.

Dr. Budson: I want to thank Chris and the panelists for sharing their personal stories and views with us. It is invaluable in our clinical and research work to see and hear from the people we are trying to help.

Index

Note: 'Page numbers followed by "f" indicate figures, "t" indicate tables and "b" indicate boxes.'

Printed and bound by CPI Group (UK) Ltd, Croydon, CR0 4YY

03/10/2024

01040385-0001